# PRACTICAL NURSING
# PHILOSOPHY

J4

04

14

004

5

TO MY GIRLS

# PRACTICAL NURSING PHILOSOPHY
## The Universal Ethical Code

David Seedhouse

*Auckland University of Technology, New Zealand*
*and Middlesex University, London, UK*

**JOHN WILEY & SONS, LTD**

*Chichester · New York · Weinheim · Brisbane · Singapore · Toronto*

*Other Wiley Editorial Offices*

John Wiley & Sons, Inc., 605 Third Avenue,
New York, NY 10158-0012, USA

WILEY-VCH Verlag GmbH, Pappelallee 3,
D-69469 Weinheim, Germany

Jacaranda Wiley, Ltd., 33 Park Road, Milton,
Queensland 4064, Australia

John Wiley & Sons (Asia) Pte, Ltd., 2 Clementi Loop #02-01,
Jin Xing Distripark, Singapore 129809

John Wiley & Sons (Canada), Ltd., 22 Worcester Road,
Rexdale, Ontario M9W ILI, Canada

*Library of Congress Cataloging-in-Publication Data*
Seedhouse, David
      Practical nursing philosophy : the universal ethical code / David Seedhouse.
         p. ; cm.
      Includes bibliographical references and index.
      ISBN 0-471-49012-1 (pbk. : alk. paper)
      I. Nursing—Philosophy.    2. Nursing ethics.    I. Title.
      [DNLM: I. Ethics, Nursing.    2. Philosophy, Nursing. WY 85 S451p 2000]
      RT84.5 .S43 2000
      610.73'01—dc21                                                     00–043437

*British Library Cataloguing in Publication Data*
A catalogue record for this book is available from the British Library

ISBN 0-471-49012-1

Typeset in 10/12pt Palatino from the author's disks by Dobbie Typesetting Limited, Tavistock, Devon
Printed and bound in Great Britain by Bookcraft (Bath) Ltd, Midsomer Norton
This book is printed on acid-free paper responsibly manufactured from sustainable forestry,
in which at least two trees are planted for each one used for paper production.

# Contents

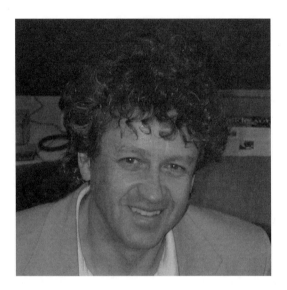

## ABOUT THE AUTHOR

**David Seedhouse** gained a doctorate in philosophy in 1984 and immediately took a post as Research Assistant in an academic nursing department. He suspected that even though philosophy is considered the most abstract of disciplines, there is nevertheless a role for philosophers prepared to take a sustained interest in practice.

The book is proof that he made the right choice. It is the culmination of fifteen years' collaboration with nurses – as observer, patient, teacher and friend – that has resulted in an unusually powerful combination of philosophical rigour and practical insight.

David is currently Professor of Health and Social Ethics at Auckland University of Technology, New Zealand, and Professor of Health Care Analysis at Middlesex University, England. He lives in Auckland with his wife, Hilary, and daughters Charlotte and Penelope.

# Foreword

This book, bold in scope, is a return to the pursuit of comprehensive nursing theory. It provides a wide-ranging, usable guide to moral behaviour in day-to-day nursing practice, and proposes a Universal Ethical Code.

*Practical Nursing Philosophy* contains important ideas for nursing ethics: it argues (against the 'ethics myth') that ethics is not just about making specific decisions but is a continual moral process.

Professor Seedhouse contends that mental health care is emblematic both of nursing's problems and its solutions. And he is right to point out that without understanding what we mean by illness, or giving due consideration to the part patients play in defining their illness, there can be little real progress in ethics.

Chapters Two to Five stand alone as an excellent exposition of concepts central to nursing and examples of how to critique and analyse them. The review of the problems with nursing's descriptions of these core concepts – advocacy, care, dignity and holism – is required reading. Each of them has, at some time or other, taken hold of nursing's collective imagination as the key concept to understanding what and who we are as nurses, but every one has fallen short of providing a single all-encompassing umbrella for nursing.

David Seedhouse poses two challenges that nursing must meet if it is to progress as a discipline. First, it must redevelop core concepts to move beyond well-meaning, but essentially emotional, expressions of ideals in order to create a specific and philosophically rigorous conceptual framework. Second, nursing should lead the way to a more humane and practical understanding of health care ethics.

Professor Seedhouse provides nursing with a template to examine our central concepts. First, he analyses the formulation of each in the nursing literature and, where necessary, condenses the expression to reveal its essence while comparing it with the conventional sense of the term. This shows the central relevance each idea has for nursing, and it also becomes apparent that none in itself can fully capture the value nurses have to offer.

The challenge is for nursing to specify concepts so they can be integrated in a way that guides the profession not only in the everyday act of giving nursing care but also in constructing rational and useful health policy. The Universal Ethical Code at the end of the book offers such a system. Each of the core concepts analysed at the beginning is integrated into a system for pragmatic guidance for the ethical practice of nursing in day-to-day interaction with patients.

Practising nursing is significantly different from practising medicine. What feels right and good about treating patients varies between nurses and physicians. Nursing gives rise to questions which just would not come up within the medical perspective.

The nature of the relationship between nurses and their patients is key to understanding the perspective nurses bring to ethics. The closeness between nurses and patients, centring around the most basic social and biological aspects of life, in addition to nurses' involvement in treatment, lends itself to endorsing David Seedhouse's contention that ethics is not about providing prescriptions for particular actions in specific dilemmas, but about the struggle to be with patients in a moral way. Thus patient care is an ethical enterprise and good nursing is synonymous with ethical nursing.

Although the content of nursing ethics is not unique, I believe that the perspective from which nurses approach questions of moral treatment is distinctive. It remains for us to turn that experience into clear moral language that is both intellectually rigorous and useful to the nurse engaged in patient care. For those of us who believe in this enterprise, the approach offered by David Seedhouse in this book is essential reading.

**Douglas P. Olsen**
**Yale University School of Nursing**

# Preface

I am not a nurse. I have never felt the daily pressure of other lives depending on what I do. But I have spent years observing nurses at work, thinking about what makes nursing important, wondering if I could help nurses do it more effectively.

I cannot write as a nurse. But I do write as one who has experienced the sometimes crushing consequences of advocating compassion in technical health systems. And I do write in support of nursing ideals, in the hope this book will make them stronger than ever.

This text is an Outsider's study of those components of nursing I can best comprehend – the philosophy, the ethics and the struggle to be heard. I offer it with respect, in the hope it might help nursing better express and apply its insights for the good of all.

The book has two aspects. It analyses nine concepts central to nursing: **advocacy**, **care**, **dignity**, **holism**, **separatism**, **research**, **ethics**, **mental health** and **nursing** itself. These analyses are contained within separate chapters, and can be read singly if necessary (perhaps by student nurses with assignment deadlines looming?).

There is also an argument running through the book, which goes like this:

There is nursing philosophy and there is analytic philosophy, and they rarely overlap. Nursing philosophy advances compassionate ideals so general 'that in explaining everything they explain nothing',[1] while analytic philosophy's dedication to intellectual purity removes it from nursing reality.

Moral conviction and logical rigour seem fixed in opposition. But combine analysis with faith in nursing values, and the ice melts. The importance of nursing's central concepts is not at issue. The question is: **what exactly do the concepts mean, and how can they be most kindly and intelligently applied?**

We know intuitively that dignity is important. But we cannot know what it is nor how to create it until we have looked to see what it is made of. Once we can see dignity's components we can work out how to foster more of it in the people we care for.

The same is true of nursing's other big ideas. It is not enough to want to advocate, care, research, be ethical and so forth. We have to understand what these ambitions consist of. Like everything else in nursing, to proceed effectively nurses need to know what they are doing, why they are doing it, and who they are doing it for.

The last two chapters unite moral commitment and logic in a hierarchy meant to encourage creative thought and practice in the cause of health. This hierarchy is condensed into a dynamic – and potentially universal – ethical code.

But the **Universal Code** does not come without a price. Some cherished beliefs do not withstand inspection. In particular, it is obvious that nursing cannot both espouse holism and claim to be a separate profession. Nor can nurses reject so-called masculine reasoning with one hand while advocating systematic research with the other.

Perhaps the most difficult conclusion to accept is that nursing values are not exclusive to nursing, and should not be promoted as such, since to do so is to perpetuate a destructive divide between different types of health carer. However, if nursing can countenance the fact that **no** profession is unique, nurses may yet take on a special role.

Nurses have nurtured values of profound moral significance. But their ideas are still not welcomed by most other health specialists. Far too much clinical work remains a mindless, tender-less pursuit of technical ends.

Of all the health professions, only nursing has the moral insight and practical wisdom to bring about general moral progress. Nursing should guard its ethical commitment no longer. Nursing should carry out and explain ethical health care in all contexts and amongst all health professions. Nursing should set out to lead by example.

**David Seedhouse**
**August 2000**

# Acknowledgements

This book has been years in the making. It has benefited from almost every conversation I have had with countless nurses, in many countries: but I must single out Leila Shotton for her unwavering support and tolerance of this project. She is the best imaginable example of a philosophical nurse.

I must also give thanks to Liverpool University (UK) – for this book really began in the late 1980s – Auckland University (NZ), Middlesex University (UK) and Auckland University of Technology (NZ). One way or another, each institution has made my research and writing possible – even enjoyable, more often than not – and I am very grateful for that.

# PART ONE

# Nursing's Big Ideas

# CHAPTER ONE

# Nursing Philosophy's Practical Failure

## SUMMARY

This chapter:

1. Outlines the theoretical and practical limitations of conventional Codes of Practice.
2. Explains why nursing philosophy fails to deliver what it could.
3. Distinguishes nursing philosophy from analytic philosophy.
4. Argues that analytic philosophy is essential if nursing philosophy's moral insights are to be converted into practical guidance for working nurses.
5. Sets the scene for the analysis of nursing's cherished concepts offered in **Chapters Two to Eight**.

◆

---

*CASE ONE*

### The Frustrated Nurse

Ann is disappointed. How she feels this morning she'd give it up now if she could. But she can't. She needs the money and there's nowhere else to go. So she fixes her lunch-box and waves him to the office. Then she shivers into her car for yet another overcrowded drive through dispiriting drizzle.

At the Residential Home she forces cheerfulness. 'I've finished the Christmas shopping at last!' 'How's little Jenny's flu?' 'He said *what?!*'

Briefly on her own, she sets out the morning's medications. But the thought's still there, however much she tries to push it out.

It's too much, we're treating them because it suits *us*. Some are slow, some are difficult, some are . . . puzzled. But that doesn't mean we should see them as *problems*. They can all be reached if we try hard enough. But we don't. *I* don't.

*continues*

_____ *continued* _____

I did once. I told the others we shouldn't do it. I said it's against our Code of Practice. It's not in the patients' interests. It's not safe to have them drowsy all the time. It's undignified.

They said it's safer because they move around less. Then they quoted passages from Codes that say nurses must behave 'professionally' and 'collaborate with colleagues'.

'Everyone else thinks the meds. are OK. There's no time and not enough staff to do even half what you want. If you can't be realistic you'd better leave.' Up to you, they said.

So I go along with it. I want to advocate but I don't know how to do it. I want to be compassionate. I want to care for them. I want to dignify them. I want us to see them for what they are – people with massive life histories. There should be a way to change it, to stand up for these elderly people, to keep them with us, to give them life. But I'm at a loss to know where to begin.

Disoriented twilight. A sly nudge from cold-hearts. A plunge into night. It's sapping me. How can it come to this in the end? How can we let it come to this?

◆

## INTRODUCTION

It is not easy to see an effective way forward for Ann. She might turn to sympathetic colleagues for support, or she could try contacting a representative of her nursing union – but otherwise she is on her own.

Neither Codes of Practice nor nursing philosophy support her sufficiently. They extol inspiring ideals: nurses should be caring, should relate to patients, should honour patient dignity, should be ethical before anything else. But they never explain how to make them real.

Take Codes of Practice. They are supposed to guide nurses in difficult situations. So why don't they help Ann?

*SECTION ONE*

## WHY NURSING CODES DON'T DELIVER

All professions* have Codes of Practice.** Some practitioners find them helpful, and they are sometimes used in disciplinary hearings – yet they are seldom more than generalities open to wide interpretation.

_____

*It matters little whether nursing is a profession or not – what matters is what nurses do.
**This chapter makes reference to three nursing Codes of Practice: the United Kingdom Central Council for Nursing, Midwifery and Health Visiting (UKCC), Code of Professional Conduct for the Nurse, Midwife and Health Visitor (3rd edition, 1992) – supplemented by the UKCC Guidelines for Professional Practice, 1996; the Canadian Nurses Association Code of Ethics for Nursing, adopted in 1985; and the Australian Nursing Council Code of Ethics for Nurses in Australia, May 1993.

# GENERAL DIFFICULTIES WITH CODES OF PRACTICE

Codes of Practice cannot provide thorough guidance because:

### 1. They must apply to all members of a profession
The tasks of a nurse working on a secure psychiatric unit are very different from those of a nurse working on a neonatal ward. A psychiatric nurse manager may have to make decisions affecting a population of thousands. A nurse working in newborn intensive care will be focussed on only a few babies (and possibly their families). Yet the nurses' Code of Practice must be sufficiently broad to advise them both.

### 2. Codes have to be acceptable to professionals from different cultural backgrounds
Codes must include all members of a profession, whatever their cultural beliefs. Therefore they must generalise. For example:

> 'A doctor must practice his profession uninfluenced by motives of profit.'[2]
> 'Nurses value the promotion of an ecological, social and economic environment which supports and sustains health and well-being.'[3]
> 'A nurse is obliged to treat clients with respect for their individual needs and values.'[4]

It might seem that doctors and nurses from any culture could subscribe to these principles, or at least not be offended by them. But even the broadest assertions do not always straddle cultural difference. Whenever something meaningful is said, the opportunity for dissent exists.

Taking the three quotes in turn: many doctors who live in cultures based on individualist values do not subscribe to the World Medical Association's enthusiasm for financial purity.[5,6]

Once the notion of a 'healthy social environment' (implicit in the Australian Nursing Council's Statement) is put into practice it is bound to include some values and exclude others – simply because spelling out what is meant must create at least one disputable opinion.[7] Ann, for instance, thinks a 'healthy social environment' implies 'rich social interactions between residents and staff' whereas her colleagues interpret it as 'quiet orderliness'.

The Canadian Code[4] claims nurses have a duty to respect all clients' 'needs and values'. However, by attempting to accommodate all values equally the statement defeats itself.

Our social world is home to countless values, not all of which are compatible. Since it asks nurses to respect **every** value, the Canadian Code inevitably requires nurses to endorse values not respected in every culture. This creates nursing problems that cannot be solved by the Code alone. For example, according to the Canadian Code nurses are obliged both to respect all people equally and to respect the values of patients who think people from other races are inferior.

### 3. Detailed Codes are Treatises
Sometimes professional Codes expand as they are discussed and revised.[8] As they do, they cover increasingly specific situations. But as soon as any Code moves from

general assertion to an argued position about what to do in particular cases it becomes a treatise (a controversial set of opinions) rather than a Code.

**It boils down to this**: if they are not to be books of moral philosophy, Codes of Practice must be short. Brief statements meant to cover all circumstances are bound to be vague. Vague statements are open to interpretation. Once interpreted, the Codes fall away – it is no longer the principles but how they are understood and applied that matters.

## WHAT ARE NURSING CODES SUPPOSED TO DO?

Nursing Codes are supposed to:

**Function A**. '...help (nurses) to reflect on the many challenges that face us in day-to-day practice'.

**Function B**. '...provide principles to aid (nurses') decision making'.

**Function C**. '...present important themes and principles which you (nurses) must apply to all areas of your work'.

(**A–C** are taken from the UKCC Guidelines for Professional Practice, 1996.)

Though Codes lend nursing a professional air, these three purposes do not hold together.

There are important differences between **fostering reflection** (**function A**), providing principles as **aids** to decision making (**function B**), and presenting principles which **must** be applied in all areas of a nurse's work (**function C**).

All aspects of life seen through curious eyes can prompt reflection (**function A**). Even rigid principles can encourage thought, but unless they are explicitly presented as starting points for intellectual analysis they are not especially likely to do so.

Whether a Code's principles are said to be **aids** (**function B**) or **principles which (nurses) must apply to all areas of (their) work** (**function C**) is no small matter. Aids and rules are different – aids may be used or not, rules are meant to be obeyed.

**Function C** may even undermine the other functions. Though it is true that instructing nurses to apply a given set of principles can make some decisions easier, an essential part of being a free-thinking professional is to be able to work things out for oneself. The truly autonomous professional can challenge assumptions, work out her own ethical stance and develop a personal philosophy of practice.

## EXAMPLES OF THE FAILURE OF NURSING CODES

**Example One: Nurses should 'promote the interests of individual patients and clients' and 'serve the interests of society'.** (UKCC Code – main statements, in emboldened preamble.)

It is not easy to establish patients' interests, and yet more difficult to balance them against broader social goals. Staff at the Residential Home interpret 'the interests of individual patients and clients' in different ways. When Ann first raised her concerns her colleagues argued that though the 'mild sedation' might not be ideal for every patient, it was in the collective interest of everyone at the Home. Left unmedicated, some patients are disruptive and loud, they said. Their uninhibited behaviour tends to unsettle and sometimes intimidate the more introverted residents. So it is better for everyone that the Home remains an orderly place.

It is not obvious who has the best case. To decide whether Ann or the others have the most ethical policy requires intellectual effort – it is not enough merely to advise nurses to 'promote patients' interests'.

### Example Two: Item 7 of the UKCC Code

Item 7 instructs nurses to:

> 7. recognise and respect the uniqueness and dignity of each patient and client, and respond to their need for care, irrespective of their ethnic origin, religious beliefs, personal attributes, the nature of their health problems or any other factor

It looks impeccably tolerant, yet reflection reveals unresolved ideological confusion.

There are **two problems. First**, 'patient' and 'client' are different notions, yet **Item 7** uses them as if they are interchangeable. Presumably this reflects nothing more than a desire to be 'politically correct'. Nevertheless, using words with different meanings as if they are identical is confusing. Different meanings have different implications: patients are vulnerable and usually need compassionate support, whereas clients are supposedly free to purchase whatever service they choose.

Certain subtleties are completely lost by conflating the two words. Dependent on her understanding of the terms, a nurse may wish to explain more to a client than she would to a patient (perhaps to convince her to buy a service, or perhaps because she reckons the client is entitled to what she has paid for). Alternatively, she may feel less need to educate her client for fear she will shop elsewhere if she learns too much about the competition.[9] Or she might nurse patients and clients in different ways because she thinks the nurse–patient relationship is potentially richer than the nurse–client relationship, which (in her opinion) can only ever be instrumental.

Whatever the case, it is a mistake to say nurses should:

> . . . recognise and respect the uniqueness and dignity of each patient and client

as if it doesn't matter what the person is called. How a person is labelled can make all the difference in the world to the way he is treated.

Ann regards the residents as clients first, patients second. Many of them are not ill – their only problem is they are old – so she feels bound to treat them with the respect she would afford any other free citizen. She also feels obliged to respond to what they want, rather than what she or the staff might want, because she is offering a contracted service. In contrast, most of her colleagues see the residents as dependent patients.

The **second problem** is that **Item 7** is incoherent. It claims each person is unique and should be treated accordingly. However, it also says that people should be cared for **irrespective** of precisely those factors which give them their uniqueness: their ethnicity, religion and personal attributes.

Presumably **Item 7**'s authors intended that nurses should deal with everyone equally whatever their problems and whatever they might think of them personally. But this isn't what the statement actually says. It tells nurses to disregard people's ethnic origin and religion, but at the same time to 'respond to their need for care' – even though it is frequently impossible to do both.

An oft-cited dilemma in health care ethics makes the problem obvious. What, according to **Item 7**, should a nurse do if a Jehovah's Witness is brought into A&E after a car crash, badly injured but conscious, and in obvious need of blood? Though shocked, he does not seem confused. He knows what's happened, that he is in a hospital, and that he needs urgent surgery. There is no time for a psychiatric assessment. He asks you to call his wife, and then says repeatedly, 'No blood, I don't want blood.' I am a Jehovah's Witness and cannot have blood. Please respect my wish.' In this case, how can the nurse possibly respect the patient's uniqueness **irrespective** of his religious beliefs?

Because of their origins, the need for care of a member of a traditional Maori or Chinese family will often be different from that of a Beverly Hills family of European descent. More than anything else, knowledge of their cultural tradition will tell the nurse how much information to give to the patient's wider family, and how much weight to give to their collective choice (usually less to the LA family and more to the non-Americans).[10]

There are **two ideologies** competing within **Item 7**: a form of individualism (respect uniqueness) and a form of socialism (treat everybody equally).[6] A Code of Practice is not the place to decide between these ideologies. But neither is it the place merely to state them without further comment. The UKCC booklet rightly acknowledges that:

> With so many codes and charters about, it is easy to be confused about how they relate to your professional and personal life. (Guidelines, p. 6)

Yet its own casual approach to philosophical analysis adds to the confusion.

*SECTION TWO*

# WHY NURSING PHILOSOPHY DOESN'T DELIVER ENOUGH

Nurse philosophers have laid claim to a moral vocabulary on nursing's behalf. Care, dignity, advocacy, ethics, health – each has been championed as the essence of nursing – yet not one of these ideas has been sufficiently worked out. Some theorists have offered 'models' of good nursing (see **Chapter Nine**), but none has been able to combine philosophical analysis, practical reasoning and moral commitment.

## NURSING'S IMPRACTICAL PHILOSOPHISING

Here are three typical examples (several others are quoted throughout this book):

**Statement 1**. 'If we did not want to care and be cared for, if we did not mind suffering and were not liable to despair or if such experiences could not be helped by companionship, then we would not need to put such a high value on caring.'[11]

**Statement 2**. '...the basic notions of caring supply a form that impulses can take which would otherwise be formless...'[11]

**Statement 3**. 'The science of human caring is indeed becoming more scientific, more human and more caring. The heart of nursing, the sensing of human need, is not only real but measurable in energy field terms.'[12]

There is no doubting the ethical enthusiasm behind such statements. The trouble is they don't say anything. Read them quickly and each sounds significant. It looks as if something important is being said. But take a step back. How profound are they really?

Most readers will feel they have some idea what is meant, and a few may even consider they understand exactly what their authors are saying. But such congruities will either be lucky guesses or illusions.

Look closely:

**Statement 1** is circular. It says nothing more than 'If we did not so much want to care and be cared for we would not want to care and be cared for so much'.

**Statement 2** is nonsense. It claims that if notions of caring did not exist then our impulses to care would be formless. But if our impulses to care really were formless we would be unable to tell we have any. It is only because we feel distinct caring emotions in the first place that we can form any concept of care at all.

**Statement 3** comes from an article that describes people as interconnected 'energy fields'. It offers an interesting way to think of the world, based very loosely on theoretical physics. It does not, however, define 'science', 'human' or 'caring'. Consequently (since there are countless alternative interpretations of these terms) it is impossible to understand the detail of what the author is trying to say, and we are left with little more than emotive gesture.

## THE PHILOSOPHY IS MISSING

Nursing is not advancing philosophically because most of its theorists confuse rhetorical assertion with substantial argument. Pick up any journal that expresses an interest in nursing philosophy and you will find pseudo-philosophical statements within minutes, if not sooner.

I am not the only one to notice that there is no chance of philosophical progress without philosophical method:

> ...nursing theorists have attempted to establish nursing as a practice discipline with its own knowledge base rather than one derived from social, biological and medical sciences...Throughout the ...literature, there is ...a recurring theme that equates nursing theory with philosophy...(but)...this derives from a colloquial understanding of philosophy and...(is) not...philosophical enquiry achieved by critical analysis of the fundamental premises on which theories rest.[13]

This point is so fundamental it bears further elucidation.

## MOST NURSING PHILOSOPHY IS NOT ANALYTIC PHILOSOPHY

Notoriously, philosophers find it hard to define what philosophy is. However, it does not follow that any sort of thinking is philosophical. Indeed, anyone who has been competently trained as a philosopher will have little difficulty distinguishing philosophically sound arguments from other sorts of reasoning.

In Western cultures, philosophy uses logic to analyse words (such as those examined in this book), arguments (of any kind), things (often commonplace objects), sensations (such as our perceptions of colour and hardness) and processes (such as scientific activity) in order to discover what makes them what they are.[14] Most philosophers accept that the results of philosophical inquiry rarely if ever tell the whole story, but nevertheless claim that the philosophical approach offers a unique insight into these subjects.

The philosophy I studied at university was in this tradition. It taught me to question assumptions – not least those I was most sure of. I learnt to reason systematically, and to dissect notions into their constituent parts in order to understand them deeply. I discovered the importance of challenging everything, and after six years had learnt enough to do it reasonably well.

Some nurse academics share this understanding of philosophy, and produce theoretically solid, practically relevant papers. But the majority confuse **insistence on favoured precepts** with **philosophical analysis**.

---

**Analytic Philosophy** (at its best)

Is done primarily in order to clarify ideas

Aims to clarify meanings before it can espouse them

Aims to produce precise definitions of key terms

Tries to minimise personal biases

---

> **Nursing Philosophy** (as a rule)
>
> Is done for purposes other than the clarification of ideas
>
> Declares its allegiance to ideas before it has thoroughly examined them
>
> Does not produce precise definitions of its key terms
>
> Promulgates 'philosophies of life' fashionable amongst a small group of nurse philosophers

*SECTION THREE*

# LOGIC AND COMMITMENT

None of the items in the 'nursing philosophy' box above are necessarily faults. We all favour imperfectly examined ideas and pursue goals we have not fully thought out. Nor does lack of definition prevent us caring. My three-year-old daughter cares for me yet she cannot explain what caring means, and I cared for my wife for years before I ever analysed the concept.

And nor is there anything wrong in principle with holding a biased philosophy of life. To nurse well one **needs** to be biased. In order consistently to work for health one must be morally committed to improving people's opportunities to flourish.

Furthermore, nursing can be special in ways that elude analysis. To nurse a stranger because she needs you can be a fundamentally moving experience. And to be nursed by a stranger – to be cared for meaningfully by someone you have never met before – is profoundly uplifting. Formal or informal, offered or received, nursing is one of the most life-giving interventions any of us can experience.

Speaking very generally, nursing is different from other types of health care because it is committed first to the pursuit of moral rather than technical ends. This distinction blurs in practice – nurses must be as technically competent as anyone else, and other health professionals can care just as deeply as nurses – nevertheless nursing has established a distinctively ethical presence.

## THE BASIC PROBLEM

But there is a problem. It is not that one sort of philosophy is right and the other wrong. Nursing philosophy's moral insight and analytic philosophy's logical rigour both have much to offer – and neither has all the answers. Rather the problem is that **too many nurse theorists are trying to force nursing philosophy to do the job only analytic philosophy can do**.

The result is that crucially important ethical notions are proclaimed, but are inadequately argued. And without substantiation they are infinitely less powerful than they should be.

## ANALYTIC AND NURSING PHILOSOPHY NEED EACH OTHER

Analytic philosophy can enhance nursing and nursing can enhance analytical philosophy. In sustained combination they could bring about a massive ethical shift in health care practice.[15]

Consider Ann's situation, for example. She has a personal understanding of what good nursing is, but can neither articulate nor apply it. She desperately wants to do the right thing, but is restricted both by her working environment and by her inability to develop her intuitions to the full. So her instincts waver between giving it all up, throwing out the medications, telling the patients what she knows, protesting to management, and contacting the newspapers.

Analytic philosophy can help. It can offer Ann (and any other health worker) the wherewithal to react with genuine feeling yet also **work out** practical ways to promote her clients' health. Ann thinks:

> Some are slow, some are difficult, some are ... puzzled. But that doesn't mean we should see them as *problems*. They can all be reached if we try hard enough. But we don't. *I* don't. I did once. I told the others we shouldn't do it. I said it's against our Code of Practice. It's not in the patients' interests. It's not safe to have them drowsy all the time. It's undignified.

But she finds she cannot convert her distress, indignation and guilt into a strategy. Yet she must if she is to bring about constructive change. She needs the insights and compassion her nursing has fostered in her, but she also needs analytic skills to decide how to make the world respond to her compassion.

It is not easy to combine moral commitment and dispassionate logic, but it is possible. For example, to say that each nurse should:

> ... respect the dignity, culture, values and beliefs of patients ...
> (The Australian Nurses' Code of Conduct 1995)

is an intuitive ethical assertion that everyone is as important as everyone else, and that nurses should act according to this principle (even if no one else will). But it does not say how Ann (or any other nurse) can **actually** respect the dignity, culture, values and beliefs of over-medicated old people.

To achieve this, analysis is essential. For example, in order for Ann to try systematically and explicitly to dignify her clients she needs to know the constituents of dignity (some people understand these intuitively, but not everyone does and not everyone understands them in the same ways, so it is necessary to spell them out).

The philosophical analysis of dignity offered in **Chapter Four** concludes:

> **If a health worker wants to promote a person's dignity she must either expand the person's capabilities or improve the person's circumstances**

Which means that the health worker must discover what a person's capabilities are, and try to create:

. . . situations where she can exercise these capabilities effectively

If this analysis is coupled with a commitment to promoting dignity there is a path forward (though of course success is not guaranteed). Armed with this definition, instead of reacting solely according to her feelings, Ann might begin to collect **evidence**. She might, for instance, put together a dossier of the patients' actual and potential capabilities (by interviewing them and, if necessary, their relatives), compile a report of the prevailing circumstances in the Rest Home, and compare and contrast the two.

The philosophical analysis of dignity provides clear practical guidance – in order to assess dignity the health worker must discover **capabilities** and match these to **circumstances**. It is not enough to say 'we aim to uphold dignity but circumstances dictate that we must medicate at present levels'. If there is a mismatch between capabilities and circumstances – and if the institution is seriously committed to promoting patient dignity – then patients must either be equipped with additional capabilities, or the institution's circumstances must be changed in order to allow patients to act freely in accord with their present capabilities.

Ann is committed to dignity, so doing nothing is not an option. But she need not act impulsively, and nor should she despair – she can use the result of the conceptual analysis of dignity to justify practical proposals for reform.

## THE LOGICAL ANALYSIS OF CHERISHED CONCEPTS

Each of the following chapters (**Two** to **Nine**) undertakes the logical analysis of cherished concepts in nursing philosophy, in order to help turn moral aspiration into practical reality. The final chapter combines the resulting definitions into a **Universal Code** that respects nurses' experience, moral insight and intelligence, acknowledges the complexity of their daily tasks, and provides a framework that allows nurses to apply the moral impulses of nursing philosophy in ways that work.

# CHAPTER TWO

# Advocacy

## SUMMARY

This chapter:

1. Distinguishes between the **normal sense** of advocacy and some **nurse theorists' sense** of advocacy.
2. Explains that the **nurse theorist sense** is too broad to be of specific help to nurses.
3. Shows that advocacy in the **normal sense** cannot be a primary nursing goal.
4. Demonstrates the ethical complexity of any decision to do something (or nothing) for another person.
5. Shows that the notion of advocacy (in either **sense**) is insufficiently powerful to guide thoughtful, creative practice.

◆

*CASE TWO*

## A Case for Advocacy?

Patricia is a forthright disciple of nurse advocacy. She sticks up for her patients whenever she can. This, she believes, is the most important job a nurse can do.

Patricia is nursing a patient called Linda, who has breast cancer. The cancer has been detected early and has not spread, so far as the scans show. The surgeon has advised conservative treatment: a lumpectomy, a course of radiotherapy, and standard check-ups afterwards.

Linda doesn't think this is enough and wants a mastectomy, radiotherapy and chemo-therapy. She has read that this is the surest way to prevent any recurrence of cancer.

Linda is desperate to get what she wants, but the surgeon refuses her request. He tells her the evidence is that a lumpectomy will be just as effective as more radical surgery and follow-up treatment, and is less damaging in other ways. If she really wants the most drastic treatment she'll have to find someone else to do it.

*continues*

---

*continued*

'Can he do this to me?' Linda asks Patricia.

'I don't know. I'm not sure. I think he's within his rights but I need to check for you. Would you like me to do that?'

'Yes please.'

Patricia takes legal advice and discovers that while Linda has a right to be treated appropriately for her condition, she does not have the right to whatever she demands. If a doctor is of the opinion that a requested treatment is not in the interest of a patient, and if he is offering therapy that a responsible body of medical practitioners would recommend, then in Western jurisdictions he is entitled to refuse.

Linda is disappointed to hear this, and does some more research of her own. She discovers that there is controversy about cancer treatment, and that different surgeons favour different policies, ranging from doing little or nothing to always doing the most thorough surgical procedure possible. She considers 'shopping around' for a different doctor, but is afraid this will eat up too much precious time, and place her in increasing danger. She also worries that once they know the story other doctors will be reluctant to go against one of their colleagues.

Patricia thinks these are very reasonable fears, and feels deeply sorry for Linda. If ever there was a case for a nurse advocate this is surely it, she thinks.

Patricia resolves to tackle the surgeon and heads off toward his office.

---

◆

---

Patricia seems to be doing the right thing. She is nursing a vulnerable woman denied a potentially life-saving treatment. She empathises with her, wants to respect her choices, and is determined to do something to improve her distressing circumstances. Yet despite its immediate appeal, Patricia's approach is not **obviously** right.

In order to assess its wisdom, several important matters need to be resolved. In what ways might her project turn out? Who might be affected? What is truly best for Linda? Does Linda have sufficient knowledge to decide for herself? Is she too anxious to reason properly? Is Patricia equipped to advocate well? Is direct action the best strategy?

*SECTION ONE*

## ADVOCACY'S DOUBLE MEANING

Before she considers these questions Patricia must decide what advocacy means. This is particularly important because there are two senses of advocacy at large: the **normal sense** and some **nurse theorists' sense**. The **normal sense** can be found in any dictionary. The **nurse theorist** sense cannot – at least not under 'advocacy'.

## THE NORMAL SENSE OF ADVOCACY

In everyday use advocacy is a simple notion:

> **An advocate speaks on behalf of some other person (or persons), as that person perceives his interests**

On this sense **an advocate supports people by taking their side directly** – this is what a legal advocate does when she argues a client's case.

An advocate in the **normal sense** cannot be impartial. She must take the part of the person for whom she is advocating. If she tries to take a balanced view, or advocates what she thinks rather than what her client wants, then she is not advocating in the **normal sense**.

## SOME NURSE THEORISTS' SENSE OF ADVOCACY

The **nurse theorist sense** of advocacy is considerably broader than the **normal** one. It means:

- **offering information to a person or persons**
- **helping a person find meaning in his illness**
- **helping a person clarify what he wants to do**

  and

- **doing things for a person that he cannot do himself**

In contrast to the **normal sense**, the **nurse theorist** understanding is that **an advocate supports people by providing, or helping them obtain, some of their basic human needs**.

Both the **normal** and the **nurse theorist** senses agree that advocates **support** other people, but the nature of this support is different. On the **normal sense** the advocate says:

> 'You're not getting what you want, would you like me to back you up as you try to get it?'

which is what Patricia wants to do for Linda. But on the **nurse theorist sense** the advocate says:

> 'You have some fundamental problems. Let me sustain you as much as I possibly can.'

The UKCC favours the latter, more expansive understanding:

Although the words advocacy and autonomy are not specifically used, it is this section (quoted below) which states the registered practitioner's role in these respects. The Code states that:

'As a registered nurse . . . you . . . must . . .

1  . . . act always in such a manner as to promote and safeguard the interests and well-being of patients and clients; (advocacy)'[16]

This is quite a claim. Giving enemas, fetching pay-phones and topping up vases usually promote patients' well-being and safeguard their interests.

Advocacy is an important concept in nursing philosophy. But are such common-place activities really 'advocacy'?

The only sure way to find out is to undertake a philosophical analysis of the **nurse theorist sense.**

# SECTION TWO

# MEANING STRETCHED TOO FAR

There is a point of view – famously advanced by Humpty Dumpty – that words can mean whatever anyone wants them to:

'I don't know what you mean by "glory",' Alice said.

Humpty Dumpty smiled contemptuously. 'Of course you don't – till I tell you. I meant "there's a nice knock-down argument for you!"'

'But "glory" doesn't mean "a nice knock-down argument",' Alice objected.

'When *I* use a word,' Humpty Dumpty said, in a rather scornful tone, 'it means just what I choose it to mean – neither more nor less.'

'The question is,' said Alice, 'whether you *can* make words mean so many different things.'

'The question is,' said Humpty, 'which is to be master – that's all.'[17]

Alice finds Humpty's argument 'unsatisfactory'. How can anyone be sure what anyone else means if words can mean anything anybody decides?

Lewis Carroll (the author of the Alice books) was aware of this objection. In an academic treatise, he wrote:

. . . I maintain that any writer of a book is fully authorised in attaching any meaning he likes to any word or phrase he intends to use. If I find an author saying, at the beginning of his book, 'Let it be understood that by the word *"black"* I shall always mean *"white"*, and that by the word *"white"* I shall always mean *"black"*,' I meekly accept his ruling, however injudicious I may think it.[18]

It is hard to disagree with Carroll. Many words have two or more meanings,[19] so it is quite possible that the **nurse theorist** sense of advocacy will become generally accepted. Yet just as we should not rewrite history at whim, Alice is surely right that there is something 'unsatisfactory' about so deliberately setting out to change the meaning of a well-established word.

## SEARCHING FOR THE BIG IDEA

In a paper frequently cited as seminal, Leah Curtin states that:

> ... the philosophical foundation and ideal of nursing is the nurse as advocate.[20]

She praises nursing 'based upon our common humanity' (an idea far removed from 'legal advocacy'):

> We are human beings, our patients or clients are human beings, and it is this commonality that should form the basis of the relationship between us.[20]

Curtin assumes that because nurses and patients have the same vulnerabilities and needs, they should form sympathetic relationships. However, the fact that human beings have common interests does not necessarily inspire moral behaviour. 'Common humanity' can be a basis for collaboration, but it is also an inexhaustible source of discord (all human conflict stems from the fact that we have similar desires).

Furthermore, 'common humanity' can be understood in contrasting ways. Some right-wingers have coined the phrase 'moral strangers' to describe people who are equally human but who do not share common moral ground.[21] For moral strangers, 'common humanity' is not a basis for caring relationships but a reason to compete – a motivation to distance yourself from human beings who do not share your moral outlook.

Curtin does not notice this rather obvious objection. She seems beguiled by the prospect of a **big idea** – a grand notion able to unite nursing's caring aspirations under a single banner. She wants advocacy to act as an umbrella for talking openly with patients and helping them find meaning. She even uses 'advocacy' to stand for 'analysis of situations' (third in the list of 'Responsibilities of Human Advocacy', below):

> Information must be provided ...
>
> 'We must – as human advocates – assist patients to find meaning or purpose in their living or in their dying. This can mean whatever the patients want it to mean ...
>
> Any application of human advocacy is subject to personal and situational interpretation by the practitioner ...
>
> Explanations and working together with a patient are not extras that nurses may choose to do, they are the essence of nursing, the essence of the nurse–patient relationship.
>
> Any application of human advocacy is subject to personal and situational interpretation by the practitioner ...[20]

Other theorists have also attempted to establish advocacy as nursing's **big idea**. Sally Gadow has gone even further than Curtin in making advocacy mean what she chooses it to.

Gadow rejects the **normal sense** altogether. Advocacy does not:

> ...consist in protecting individuals' *right* to do what they want. [Advocacy] is the effort to help persons *become clear about what they want* to do, by helping them discern and clarify their values in the situation, and on the basis of that self-examination, to reach decisions which express their reaffirmed, perhaps recreated, complex of values.[22]

In short, nurse advocates should assist patients:

> ...to authentically exercise their freedom of self-determination.[22]

All of which means (rather bizarrely) that Gadow's 'existential advocate' will help people work out what they want, but will not help them get it.

Elizabeth Arnold also loses control of meaning as she discusses advocacy. In her opinion:

> Advocacy involves actions taken on behalf of the patient when he or she cannot perform them.[23]

Arnold's definition is partly in keeping with the **normal sense** – traditionally an advocate acts for someone when that person either can't argue for herself, or can't argue her case as effectively as the advocate. But as Arnold has it, the phrase means rather more than this.

Consider a simple illustration:

> Molly Smith is confined to her hospital bed. She wants to pay a cheque into her bank urgently, but cannot visit the bank herself. She asks the nurse if she'd mind doing it. The nurse agrees and pays in the cheque.

The nurse does something on behalf of a patient who cannot do it herself. So what has happened? Has advocacy occurred, or has a nurse been kind and dropped a cheque into a bank?

Even when she uses examples that ought logically to lead to the conclusion that it is nonsense to claim so much for advocacy, Arnold is undeterred:

> The final exemplar of this important aspect of caring in nursing practice may seem a little strange, but *it serves to personify the nurse as the patient's advocate* in the broadest sense. The patient had just died and the student relates:
>
>> As Sandy and I were beginning to put her in the bag, Sandy's care continued. She kept the patient's modesty intact by keeping her covered with a gown. She took a washcloth and wiped Mrs S.'s face...[23]
>
> (My italics – note how Arnold admits that extending the meaning of advocacy is a deliberate ploy.)

This is surely more than 'a little strange'. The thoughtful nurse is not keeping Mrs S.'s 'modesty intact' (or preserving her dignity – see **Chapter Four**) because Mrs S. isn't there anymore. And if she is advocating for her then advocacy surely stands for 'every desirable nursing practice'.

This is not to say that these kindnesses are unimportant. Nurses certainly should perform many actions:

> . . . on behalf of the patient when he or she cannot perform them.

But it is playing with words to insist they are all 'advocacy'.

## THE BIG IDEA MAKES THINGS WORSE

There is no mistaking the enthusiasm of nurse philosophy's search for the 'foundational concept of nursing', but it is a blind alley. And not only does the pursuit of the **big idea** hit a wall, it makes matters worse.

Here's the problem:

1. **Opting for one 'foundational notion' means that useful, separate meanings and actions are substituted by one non-specific, general term.**
2. **Trying to make one word encapsulate so much makes that word superfluous.**
   Assume advocacy means what Leah Curtin says it does. Now imagine giving directions to a bus station using a stranger's map. You 'provide information' (the bus station is here), give 'an explanation' (here's how to get from here to there), and 'work together' with the stranger (let's go through the route on your map). But there is no plausible reason whatsoever to rename your already adequately labelled behaviours 'advocacy'.
3. **Going for the big idea leaves practising nurses floundering, without a framework on which to construct thoughtful practice.**
   Without detailed analyses of the applications of each **big idea**, working nurses can do no more than guess at nurse philosophers' practical advice. If advocacy can mean so much, the responsibility to interpret it must rest on nurses in the field. To instruct a nurse to advocate when advocacy can mean almost anything is no more help than telling her to be good.

There are books and journals full of different forms of advocacy. For example, Andrew Crowden[24] identifies six 'types' of advocacy: legal, individual, systemic, informal, formal and social. But these are merely descriptions of the ways anyone might advocate for other people in different circumstances. They do not provide a framework for reflection.

## EXCELLENT MOTIVE, POOR DELIVERY

None of this is to disagree with nurse philosophers' general understanding of nursing (indeed, their basic ideas are similar to the **foundations theory of health** summarised in **Chapter Eight**). The trouble is, their musings render nursing mysterious when they ought to be making it clearer.

**In sum**, nurse theorists ought not to re-classify advocacy in order to claim it as nursing's own: **firstly** because advocacy is not unique to nursing, and **secondly** because straightforward words already exist for all the actions the theorists want to re-label.

SECTION THREE

## HOW ANALYTIC PHILOSOPHY CAN HELP

Should a nurse do anything a patient asks? Should she help a paraplegic end his life if that's what he asks of her? Should she transcribe a vicious letter from an unhappy patient to a husband she blames for her misfortune? Should she give the information a patient asks for or give what she thinks a patient needs, if these are different? Should she give information she knows will confuse or alarm a patient? What if a person finds a negative meaning in his illness? Should the 'nurse advocate' continue to help her patient explore it? Or should she help the patient find only positive meanings?

Why should nurses advocate (in either **sense**)? Why should nurses help people clarify their goals? Why should they help them make decisions? Why should they help them see through their decisions? Should they do this in every case or are there times when it is better to do something else? To what extent should a nurse influence a patient's value clarification? Should she counsel, should she facilitate without directing, should she merely offer information, should she help the patient work through it, should she educate, should she say what she would do? Should she ever pressure a patient to change his mind?

All these questions require much more than a commitment to advocacy. In the first place, they need analysing.

## WHY ADVOCACY IS NOT ENOUGH

Every nursing situation – however commonplace – is potentially ethically complex. Nurses owe it to themselves and their patients to think beyond the **big ideas**.

## THERE IS NO SUBSTITUTE FOR CAREFUL THINKING

The following analysis demonstrates why it is always unwise to advocate without sustained thought. It reflects the complications any competent, caring professional must assess. It is based on the **normal sense** of advocacy (which is how most nurses understand the term):

Practising nurses ... tend to define advocacy in fairly simple terms. For example:
'*An advocate is* someone *who stands up for the patient and kind of watches out for the patient; intervenes with physicians and looks out for patients' personal wants and desires'* or '*It means protecting and defending a patient's best interests as defined by the patient or their family'.*[25]

A more extensive analysis would be necessary if the **nurse theorist sense** were used.

## SHOULD PATRICIA ADVOCATE FOR LINDA? AN ELEMENTARY PHILOSOPHICAL ANALYSIS

Generally speaking, in order to decide whether to advocate a nurse might speculate:

'I shall advocate (in the **normal sense**) for Patient X IF she ...'

and then select one of the categories **A–P*** in order to finish the phrase.

(*Note: for ease of reference the list below is divided into **3 sets**:

- **The patient has adequate knowledge and has reasoned competently**
- **The patient has inadequate knowledge and has reasoned competently**
- **The patient has reasoned incompetently**

There are combinations of possibilities within each set. The emboldened type indicates phrases that have changed from the previous combination.)

## THE ANALYSIS

Here are the possibilities facing Patricia:

'I shall advocate (in the **normal sense**) for Linda IF she ...'

---

## COMBINATIONS A–D

## HAS ADEQUATE KNOWLEDGE AND HAS REASONED COMPETENTLY

**A.** 1. has adequate knowledge
2. has reasoned competently
3. there is no conflict with others' interests
4. I agree with her decision

_____ *continues* __

— *continued* —

**B.** 1. has adequate knowledge
2. has reasoned competently
3. there is no conflict with others' interests
4. **I disagree with her decision**

**C.** 1. has adequate knowledge
2. has reasoned competently
3. **there is conflict with others' interests**
4. **I agree with her decision**

**D.** 1. has adequate knowledge
2. has reasoned competently
3. there is cónflict with others' interests
4. **I disagree with her decision**

The question for Patricia is, **which of these groups A–D (if any) most accurately represents the actual situation? Which (if any) should she insert to complete the phrase?**

---

◆

---

# COMBINATIONS E – H

# HAS INADEQUATE KNOWLEDGE AND HAS REASONED COMPETENTLY

**E.** 1. **has inadequate knowledge (false or incomplete beliefs)**
2. has reasoned competently
3. **there is no conflict with others' interests**
4. **I agree with her decision**

**F.** 1. has inadequate knowledge
2. has reasoned competently
3. there is no conflict with others' interests
4. **I disagree with her decision**

**G.** 1. has inadequate knowledge
2. has reasoned competently
3. **there is conflict with others' interests**
4. **I agree with her decision**

**H.** 1. has inadequate knowledge
2. has reasoned competently
3. there is conflict with others' interests
4. **I disagree with her decision**

The question for Patricia is, **which of these groups E–H (if any) most accurately represents the actual situation? Which (if any) should she insert to complete the phrase?**

# COMBINATIONS I–P

# HAS REASONED INCOMPETENTLY

I.  1. **has adequate knowledge**
    2. **has reasoned incompetently**
    3. **there is no conflict with others' interests**
    4. **I agree with her decision**

J.  1. has adequate knowledge
    2. has reasoned incompetently
    3. **there is conflict with others' interests**
    4. I agree with her decision

K.  1. has adequate knowledge
    2. has reasoned incompetently
    3. there is no conflict with others' interests
    4. **I disagree with her decision**

L.  1. has adequate knowledge
    2. has reasoned incompetently
    3. **there is conflict with others' interests**
    4. I disagree with her decision

M. 1. **has inadequate knowledge**
    2. has reasoned incompetently
    3. **there is no conflict with others' interests**
    4. **I agree with her**

N.  1. has inadequate knowledge
    2. has reasoned incompetently
    3. **there is conflict with others' interests**
    4. I agree with her

O.  1. has inadequate knowledge
    2. has reasoned incompetently
    3. **there is no conflict with others' interests**
    4. **I disagree with her**

P.  1. has inadequate knowledge
    2. has reasoned incompetently
    3. **there is conflict with others' interests**
    4. I disagree with her

The question for Patricia is, **which of these groups I–P (if any) most accurately represents the actual situation? Which (if any) should she insert to complete the phrase?**
(Note that if **P** pertains it is surely safe to assume that a nurse ought **not** to advocate in the **normal sense**.)

## ILLUSTRATION

Consider **combination A** first. It looks like this:

'I (**Linda**) shall advocate (in the **normal sense**) for **Patricia** IF she . . .' **A**
1. has adequate knowledge
2. has reasoned competently
3. there is no conflict with others' interests
4. I agree with her decision.'

This is the ideal combination for advocacy in the **normal sense**, however it remains for Patricia to confirm that it **most accurately represents the actual situation**.

Patricia is devoted to advocacy in the **normal sense**, so she is about to confront the surgeon who will not do the operation Linda wants. But, on the evidence available, Patricia cannot yet be certain that **A** is the most accurate representation.

She has instinctively sided with Linda, and enthusiastically checked out the law for her. Patricia can see that Linda is terrified and wants to do what she can to ease her fear. However, Patricia has not established the extent of Linda's **knowledge** (which books did she read? How old are they? Did she understand them correctly?) and nor has she established whether her patient has **reasoned competently** (what effect has her psychological state had on her thinking?). She also knows there is at least a *prima facie* **conflict with others' interests** (the surgeon doesn't want to do something damaging, and Patricia has no idea what Linda's family thinks).

**Furthermore**, Linda needs to clarify the notions **adequate knowledge**, **competent reasoning**, and **conflict with others' interests**. She does not have to do this in every case – but she must form a **considered general view** in order to make sound decisions.

To take each expression in turn:

1. **Adequate and Inadequate Knowledge**
   Not only does Linda need to know what counts as adequate knowledge, she must also establish who should decide.

a. **What Should Count as Adequate Knowledge?**
   To answer this question one must establish who it is that knows and what it is they need the knowledge for, since what counts as 'adequate' can vary enormously depending on circumstances. Adequate knowledge for a new-born baby is that his mother will feed him when he cries (that is all he needs to know). At the other extreme, it is impossible even to specify what sort of knowledge would be adequate for scientists trying to understand dolphin language (we do not yet know, for instance, whether dolphins have a language, or if they do whether it is accessible to human understanding).

   Even if there is general agreement about what level of knowledge is adequate in nursing situations, there may nevertheless be disagreement about what is adequate in particular cases.

   For example, does Linda need to know about all forms of cancer in order to make a decision about breast cancer? Is it necessary that she knows the extent to which the experts disagree about resection? To what extent does she need to understand probability theory and statistics? How many pictures of the results of mastectomies and lumpectomies does she need to see in order to grasp the reality of what might happen? How many fellow patients does she need to meet before she is sufficiently informed of the social and emotional implications of her choice?

There is also a question about what counts as adequate knowledge for Patricia. If she is not up-to-date with the latest breast cancer treatments she may find it difficult to assess the material Linda has been reading, and will not be in the best position to challenge the surgeon.

### b. Who Should Decide What Counts as Adequate Knowledge?

Who should say what level of knowledge is 'adequate'? Should it be the clinical staff? Should it be Linda? Should it be Linda even though she knew nothing about cancer four weeks ago? Should it be Linda even though she is under extraordinary pressure at the moment?

Patricia has various options. The two most obvious are that she might assume either **i** or **ii** below:

### i. Knowledge Means True Beliefs

One either has knowledge or not – strictly speaking there are no half measures. If a person believes what is true, then she knows. If she believes what is false, she doesn't. If a patient thinks a radical mastectomy offers a 95% prospect of survival after 5 years and the fact is that it offers only a 50% chance the patient has a false belief, and so does not have knowledge.

If she chooses this understanding of knowledge then Patricia might decide not to advocate until she is sure Linda has true beliefs.

### ii. Adequate Knowledge is at Least That Which the Nurse Would Require Were She the Patient

This option is less strict than **i**, but is complicated by the fact that different health workers require different depths of belief when they are patients themselves. Some want to know everything there is to know, others are content to let others decide things for them[26] – and there is every position in between. Yet **ii** is not a bad rule of thumb because most health workers will have sound knowledge in any case, and will know where to find out more if they need it.

### 2. Competent/incompetent Reasoning

What counts as competent and incompetent reasoning is as arguable as what counts as knowledge. There is a branch of philosophy (logic) devoted to the study of good reasoning. For a logician the content of a person's argument is (in most cases) irrelevant – what matters is its structure or form. This structure can be either valid or not, dependent on whether it conforms to the rules of logical argument.

There are many helpful works available on this topic – some designed specifically for health professionals.[27,28] It is not necessary to be an expert logician to be a nurse. However, a nurse trying to decide whether or not to advocate in **the normal sense** must – at the very minimum – ask: **does this patient's reasoning process make sense?** Are there any contradictions in it? Is it consistent with the patient's thinking about other matters? Does he use the same reasons every time he explains his position? If not, are the different sets of reasons compatible?

In addition to logic, there are matters of content to consider. The nurse must decide whether the **basis** of a person's reasoning makes sense. How convincing are her reasons for her decision?

There are, for instance, important differences between a patient deciding to do something on the basis of a Tarot card reading, because the surgeon has red hair and she doesn't trust redheads, because she has been advised by a leading clinician in the field, because her father wants her to, because she is herself a leading clinician in the field, because she has spent a week in the library researching the area, or because she doesn't mind whether she lives or dies. The nurse needs to consider whether her reasons are good, bad or indifferent before she agrees to help her patient get what she wants.

### 3. Others' Interests

The relevance of other people's interests varies from case to case. Are the others patients on the same ward, other patients competing for a scarce resource, relatives, other members of the public, or staff ? Whoever they are, the nurse should consider: to what extent will advocating for the patient damage their interests? Do the others have a legitimate point of view on the matter? Who says? Is anyone advocating this point of view on their behalf?

These questions also require serious thought. To reflect on them, the nurse analyst might first set up this hypothesis:

> **My advocacy for this patient will be detrimental to the interests of** ... **X, Y, Z** ... (Naming and identifying those who will be affected)

If she does not know who else might be affected then she would be wise to find out before advocating.

She might then continue:

> **In this case the interests of this other person/these other people are** ... **A, B, C** ... (Identifying what they actually are)

And then state:

> **These interests are** .........................

And fill in the dots with:

> i. **Trivial**
> ii. **Of less importance than my patient's**
> iii. **Of equal importance to my patient's**
> iv. **Of more importance than my patient's**

If she chooses **i** or **ii** then the nurse might feel justified in proceeding with her advocacy in **the normal sense**, if **iv** she ought to stop unless she is committed to **blind advocacy** (advocacy in the **normal sense** whatever the circumstances) and if **iii** she will need to think further. Perhaps she is advocating for a scarce resource – say a dialysis service – which another patient needs just as much. In such a situation, a further justification is required. Why isn't she advocating for the other patient (if there is only one other party with an interest)? Why not for both of them? And why not for all dialysis patients?

## PATRICIA NEEDS TO DO MORE WORK BEFORE SHE TACKLES THE SURGEON

It may be that:

**A. 4.** The nurse agrees with the patient's decision

instantly and intuitively (as Patricia does). However, on its own this is not a good reason to proceed. Indeed, it may be a bad one in so far as it prevents proper assessment of points **A 1–3**. Does Linda:

1.  have adequate knowledge?
2.  exhibit competent reasoning?

Is there:

3.  conflict with others' interests?

These matters need to be checked out. If **1** and **2** are true, and if there is no conflict with others' interests, then there is a good case for advocacy in the **normal sense**.

**In sum**, even the above fairly basic discussion of **combination A** indicates the extent of reasoning needed for a nurse to make a reasonable decision in an unremarkable case like Linda's.

Now consider **combination B**:

I shall advocate (in the **normal sense**) for Patient X IF:

1.  she has adequate knowledge
2.  she has reasoned competently
3.  there is no conflict with others' interests
4.  **I disagree with her decision**

For the sake of elucidation, imagine slightly changed circumstances. Imagine Patricia thinks Linda is making a mistake. Should she now advocate for her in the **normal sense**?

Imagine Patricia is satisfied that Linda has sufficient information, has thought it through well, and no one else has an interest in the matter – yet she feels intensely that Linda will regret the mastectomy. Patricia can't put her fears fully into words – they are the product of twenty years' experience of nursing breast cancer – but she has a profound instinct that Linda will react badly to the results of the operation. Patricia genuinely cares for Linda and thinks it would be uncaring not to try to get the happiest result for her.

In this case, by pleading the cause of the patient, Patricia would be casting aside years of seasoning as a nurse – disregarding her apprehensions and wisdom – for the sake of **blind advocacy**. Patricia might eventually be justified in advocating for Linda in the **normal sense** on **combination B**, but only after doing other things first. At the very least Patricia would have to try to convey her anxieties to Linda, to say she thinks she is making a mistake, to talk with Linda about what she read in the library, to see whether she interprets it properly, and to set out the pros and cons as fully as possible.

To do these other things would – of course – be to advocate in the **nurse theorist sense**. But deeper thought and skill are required to do this responsibly.

If Linda remains adamant, if she feels increasingly pressured, and if Patricia is the only person in a position to support her, then she might possibly be right to advocate for her in the **normal sense** – even though she disagrees.

## A–P ARE MORE THAN SUBTLE VARIATIONS

It should by now be plain that the combinations **A–P** are not just subtle variations. In fact, even if only one factor changes the nurse's deliberation can – and sometimes must – alter radically.

**Combination C**, for instance, differs from **A** – the ideal – only at **3**. Yet its effect is to force the nurse to reflect much more deeply about her position than she has to under **combination A**.

For illustration, consider a case in which a patient comes to you (a practice nurse) to ask you to advocate on her behalf to her doctor. She has made a study of the literature on childhood immunisation and has decided, on balance, that she will not have her infant son vaccinated. Her doctor is not happy with this decision, and has told her – in no uncertain terms – that she is being irresponsible. Should you advocate for her?

As always, there is a need to think carefully. Even if you share the mother's point of view this does not necessarily mean that you should speak on her behalf. You might, for instance, be unreasonably biased. Or the consequences might be bad for you, if you take a patient's side against a doctor. Or you might decide that other people's interests take precedence in this particular case (perhaps you work in a disadvantaged area and you are getting closer and closer to 'herd immunity' – you can see the wider picture, even though you would want what the mother wants if you were her).

None of the four considerations is necessarily compelling. For example, consider **combination D** with reference to the immunisation case. All the details are as before – the only difference is you disagree with the mother.

However, your point of view is but one of several factors in the case. Even though you think she is wrong, and even though you might damage yourself and the drive to achieve 'herd immunity', there may still be grounds to advocate **in the normal sense** for the worried mother. She may be at the end of her tether, she may be desperate for **someone** to take her side in otherwise overwhelming circumstances, and there is a good chance she may not visit the surgery again for any reason if she perceives the whole practice as intransigent.

## FLOW CHART A

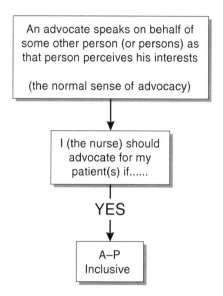

An advocate speaks on behalf of some other person (or persons) as that person perceives his interests

(the normal sense of advocacy)

I (the nurse) should advocate for my patient(s) if......

YES

A–P
Inclusive

**Figure I**  Irresponsible advocacy

## FLOW CHART B

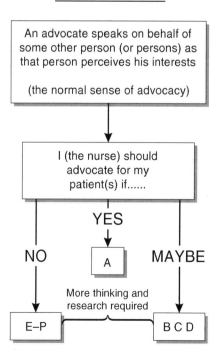

An advocate speaks on behalf of some other person (or persons) as that person perceives his interests

(the normal sense of advocacy)

I (the nurse) should advocate for my patient(s) if......

YES

NO        A        MAYBE

More thinking and research required

E–P        B C D

**Figure 2**  Thoughtful advocacy, requiring more powerful health work notions

## A NURSE'S OBLIGATIONS ARE NEITHER SIMPLE NOR SIMPLISTIC

It should by now be obvious that advocacy as described (in either sense) by nurse theorists and Codes is not on its own enough to help a nurse decide what to do – a deeper and more powerful idea is needed.

It is plainly inadequate to say:

> **The nurse is obligated to advocate the client's interest**

or any like expression. The nurse is not obliged to do this – not even using advocacy in the **normal sense**.

The simple flow charts depicted in **Figures 1** and **2** show how unrealistic it is to suggest that the nurse is obliged to advocate in the **normal sense**:

If you believe that:

> **An advocate should speak on behalf of some other person (or persons), as that person perceives his interests**

**regardless of any other considerations** then you must act according to **FLOW CHART A**. That is, you will advocate in the **normal sense** for your client whatever he does or does not know, however he has arrived at his decision, whether or not your advocacy will be counter to the interests of others, and whether or not you agree with him. But to do this as a rule would be nothing less than irresponsible.

If you believe that:

> **An advocate should speak on behalf of some other person (or persons), as that person perceives his interests**

but advocacy is governed by more important health work notions then you will act according to **FLOW CHART B** (or some similar version). You might – in the end – advocate in the **normal sense**, but you must first achieve significant other goals.

## CONCLUSION

Neither advocacy in the **normal** nor **nurse theorist sense** is enough on its own. The **normal sense** requires that a nurse speak on behalf of the patient, but in order to do this she must first decide which of the **combinations A–P** pertain, and comprehend how they represent the actual situation. And she needs more than devotion to advocacy to do this.

The **nurse theorist sense** requires that the nurse gives broader support to the patient – perhaps helping her clarify what she feels and helping her make autonomous decisions. However, not only is this a far-fetched and confusing extension of advocacy's meaning, it is also prone to the same difficulty as the **normal sense**. That is, the nurse needs to work out how and to what extent to support the patient – and to do this she needs more than a commitment to advocacy. She needs a reasoned and justified understanding of nursing's purpose.

# CHAPTER THREE

# Care

## SUMMARY

This chapter:

1. Notes that most nurse theorist writing on care is theoretically weak and therefore impractical.
2. Offers a **general definition of care**.
3. Identifies and illustrates **four types of caring**.
4. Explains why **care cannot be the most fundamental nursing principle**.
5. Shows that **caring theory** alone is not enough to help nurses decide what sort of care to provide in practical situations.

—————————— ◆ ——————————

*SECTION ONE*

## INTUITION IS NOT ENOUGH

Most nurse theorists assume that nursing:

> ... has a well-articulated philosophy of care ...[29]

Many are of the opinion that:

> Human care ... is gradually replacing a preoccupation with medical ethics that is focussed on diseases ... [N]urse care scholars ... have contributed to this world-wide cultural movement to make human care knowledge ... one of the most significant developments in the history of nursing ... human care with a transcultural focus will be nursing's unique discipline contribution to humanity.[30]

However, though care is perhaps the biggest **big idea** in nursing philosophy, it is not the robust concept the theorists think it is.

According to **caring theory**:

> Caring in nursing is a holistic construct made apparent in nursing practice as a virtue through nurses' actions and attitudes, which are reflected by the deep knowledge they have of themselves as committed caregivers.[31]

The author of this quote illustrates her understanding of care by citing an interview with the nurse of a mother of nine-month-old twins:

> Beside teaching her about the normal baby's development and her babies, I'm also teaching her about her own growth and development as a mother and as a person. I'm giving her emotional support; I'm reassuring her that life will go on, the children will grow up, and this is why we're planning. I let her know she is doing a good job . . . touching and playing with the babies, reviewing the schedule with her assists her to maintain a schedule with two individual babies. Everything was caring, visiting her, being supportive to her. Earlier in the relationship, there was more concrete teaching: this is the way you bathe, dress, etc. . . .[31]

This nurse undoubtedly provided kind and thoughtful help to the mother. But the theoretical relationship between what she did and:

> . . . a holistic construct made apparent in nursing practice as a virtue through nurses' actions and attitudes, which are reflected by the deep knowledge they have of themselves as committed caregivers[31]

is at best obscure.

Why is care a 'holistic construct'? Does the reference to 'holism' mean that every nursing practice is caring? Who has constructed the 'construct', and why? What is this 'deep knowledge' nurses have of themselves? How is it different from the knowledge anyone else has of herself?

Unless such questions are answered we cannot know what care is, other than by intuition. And without a non-intuitive explanation it is impossible to check whether nurses (and nurses and patients) have the same understandings of care.

Moreover, intuition (however deeply felt) is rarely enough to deal constructively with the practical difficulties of trying to help others in our complicated social world. Generally speaking, it may be the case that:

> To care for another person, in the most significant sense, is to help him grow and actualize himself. Consider, for example, a father caring for his child. He respects the child as existing in his own right and as striving to grow. He feels needed by the child and helps him grow by responding to his need to grow. Caring is the antithesis of simply using the other person to satisfy one's own needs.[32]

But whenever we wish to care practically for someone else we face a question that forces us beyond the limits of intuition: **how should I care for this person in these circumstances?**

**How** should a father care for his child when his striving to grow means he is consistently aggressive toward his mother? **How** should a father respond to his son's stated need for independence when he is certain his son is not yet ready for such responsibility? Must a caring father help his daughter grow in the direction she wants even if it devastates him emotionally to see her pursue her life choices?

Most leading nurse philosophers appreciate that **caring theory** must somehow connect with **caring practice**:

...caring is a value and an attitude that has to become 'a will, an intention, or a commitment' that 'manifests itself in concrete acts'[33]

But the temptation to mystify seems to overwhelm them:

Benner and Wrubel, and Benner, in seeking to make what was invisible more visible, emphasize the primacy of caring as a basic way of being in the world – that emphasizes what matters. Noddings links caring to the feminine spirit, the eros, as contrasted with the masculine spirit, the logos. Gadow, myself and others posit caring as a moral ideal that guides and directs human actions, not just as a means, but a human end in and of itself that is of intrinsic value to human civilization. A critical point is that these values and views of woman and caring are not just woman values, but values for all humanity.

Like Walker, French, Benner, Noddings and others such as Leininger, Ray, Gaylin and Mayeroff, I, too, link caring to the survival of humanity... If caring is to be sustained, those who care must be strong, courageous, and capable of inner love, peace and joy – both in relation to themselves and others.[34]

If caring is:

...a moral ideal that guides and directs human actions, not just as a means, but a human end in and of itself that is of intrinsic value to human civilization[34]

we need to be told what it is and how we can apply it to bring about helpful practical change. Otherwise we gain nothing whatsoever from reading about it.

Since not everyone acts according to 'woman values' (if we did there would be no point in writing about them) they must be explained. And the way to explain them (if they can be explained) is to encounter them, demonstrate them, or describe them. Whatever the case, theoretical distinctions (at the very least between 'woman values' and 'other values') must be made or we are left in the dark.

But care need not be an obscure notion, as the following section explains.

SECTION TWO

# FOUR TYPES OF CARING

## A. THE VIEW THAT CARING IMPLIES EMOTIONAL INVOLVEMENT

The closest the advocates of caring theory come to explaining **how** nurses should care is to suggest that if a person is to care properly for another she should be 'emotionally involved with' him.

In Jean Watson's opinion caring is:

...inspired by a yearning for the good... it is not just an emotion, concern, or a benevolent desire... It is not just knowledge; wisdom beyond knowledge is necessary to understand the individual's subjective life – world of suffering.[35]

According to Watson, in order to care for someone the carer must 'understand the individual's subjective life'. She must be:

> ...touched by human suffering[36]

in a profound way.[37] In similar vein Noddings thinks care:

> ...involves a kind of indwelling relationship, an engrossment and motivational displacement derived from feminine emotional qualities. The carer finds her true self when she chooses to become involved in caring relationships.[38]

To care like this a carer needs more than competence and kindness, she must be devoted to her patients. Marilyn Ray makes this requirement quite explicit. In her opinion:

> ...caring...[involves]...a process of co-presence, giving, receiving, communication, and in essence loving in the sense that Marcel conveyed; that is, oblative love or other-directedness.[39]

'Oblative love' is essentially a religious term. Even in the non-religious sense an oblation is an offering or a gift presented unconditionally. Yet this is too much to ask of most personal relationships, never mind professional ones.

The majority of nurses realise this, of course, and tend to be careful about how much they care. Most feel and express emotional involvement with at least some of their patients, but appreciate how important it is to avoid over-commitment.

The 'emotional involvement' concept is no help to the nurse who wants to know: does my loving this woman patient mean I should agree to everything she asks of me? Does it mean I should not give her baby daughter a life-saving blood transfusion because she forbids it? And if it does, how can I care coherently for both mother and daughter? How can I love them equally? Nor can 'emotional caring' offer a solution to the nurse who asks: how should I choose between my patients when I cannot help them all? And nor does it offer anything to the nurse who has to care for the mass murderer with second-degree burns, whom she cannot possibly bring herself to love.

The unqualified advocacy of the position that 'you must be emotionally involved to care' obscures the practicalities. Personal involvement with patients is undoubtedly an important and undervalued part of health care, but it does not guarantee good outcomes.

## A DEFINITION OF CARE

The only responsible way to advise others to care is to define your terms. And it is not difficult to define **care** and **caring**.

Conventionally, care can be used either as a noun – as in 'to have a care' (to have an object or matter of care which requires attention) – or as a verb (as in 'to care'). Thus – merely from observing the common use of language – it is possible to propose that:

**In order to care a person must have a concern for something or somebody (she must have an object of care and some interest in it)**

## EMOTIONAL INVOLVEMENT IS NOT ALWAYS NECESSARY IN ORDER TO CARE

According to this definition I can care for my daughters, my garden and my bicycle, but I do not necessarily have to have an emotional involvement to do so. I do have an emotional involvement with my daughters of course, and I have quite a passion for my garden, but even so I can, at times, meaningfully care for both without 'engrossment' and 'self-actualisation'. Sometimes, when I read Charlotte a story or give Penny a cuddle while I'm thinking about something else, or when I'm potting plants or cleaning my bike when I would rather be out having a beer, I am caring without emotional commitment.

Importantly, if care is as defined above, then meaningful health care can be done without direct emotional involvement, as follows.

## B. CARING AS PERFORMING CONVENTIONAL ACTIVITIES OF CARE

Given that a person is prepared to carry out those activities which conventionally constitute 'caring for a sick person', it is possible for her to care automatically, without having any feeling of involvement with the person being cared for. In this case the carer's emotional state is irrelevant to her caring.

Practical caring without emotional attachment is an everyday fact of nursing life – it happens whenever health care is regarded as a job of work to be performed competently. For example:

> Graham moves around the ward absentmindedly puffing pillows, speaking standard words of comfort, and checking to see that patients are stable. He does this every day because this is what is expected of him and it has become his habit.

Graham is clearly not exercising 'wisdom beyond knowledge', but he is nevertheless caring because he has an interest in doing these standard tasks properly – they are his 'objects of care'.

## IT IS POSSIBLE TO CARE WITH NEGATIVE FEELINGS

It would be possible for Graham to care with negative feelings. It does not over-extend the notion of care (as defined above) to say that one person can care for another whom she dislikes.

For example:

Simone is a widow of 52. It has fallen to her to care for Deirdre, her mother-in-law (also widowed), who suffers from Alzheimer's disease. Her tasks, which she performs efficiently, out of a sense of duty to her late husband, are to keep Deirdre clean, fed, comfortable and safe from harm. Simone found Deirdre unpleasant even when she was well, deeply resents having to do these things for her, and wishes Deirdre would die.

It would plainly be wrong to say that Simone cares for Deirdre in the sense of being positively emotionally attached to her, yet it is hard to see how it can plausibly be said that she is not caring for her mother-in-law (she has an object of care – in this case Deirdre – and an interest in caring – her sense of duty). Even if she were a desperately unhappy witness to the decline of a much-loved relative, it would be practically impossible for her to offer any greater degree of practical care than she is doing already.

## C. CARING AS BEING PRUDENT

An associated sense of caring is to care by exhibiting those actions most likely to be productive. This does not necessarily require a direct personal interest in another person either. For example:

Dorothy, a senior midwife, is called into a delivery room as complications arise. She uses her skills and experience appropriately, and saves the day. Dorothy has never spoken to the mother, and never will.

The midwife is not emotionally connected to her patient in any sense other than that she knows she is a human being in distress. Nevertheless it would be nonsense to say she is not caring for her. Dorothy is prudently offering technical care by performing those activities which she has taken the trouble to identify as being the most conducive to a successful outcome.

These two senses – caring as performing conventional activities and caring as being prudent – are almost always associated. But **they are not necessarily related** since it is possible for prudence to override tradition in exceptional circumstances (for instance, where a patient might suffer harm if a nurse were to perform a routine task thoughtlessly, or where the routine task would be damaging).

## D. PORTRAYING CARING

It is also possible to care by portraying a personal interest in someone, in order to bring about a desired result, even though the carer does not actually feel an attachment. For example:

Melanie is having a hard time at home. She usually works nights, and rarely manages to spend long with her husband. Partly as a result of this her marriage is rapidly deteriorating. She is sad and anxious about this state of affairs, and feels utterly emotionally drained. She cannot think for long about anything else.

However, Melanie knows she must keep her job as a nurse, and knows too that many patients respond better to those nurses who show a personal interest in them. Consequently, she decides to behave as much as possible as she normally would – she is pleasant and seems very interested in the affairs of her patients, even though she actually has to reserve all her emotional energy to cope with her own situation.

Portraying caring is one of a raft of professional skills, and is presumably commonplace. Caring in this sense is akin to the kind of hospitality provided by some airline stewards. It is not necessarily false, but it is likely to be false at least sometimes. And so long as the passenger does not notice the falsehood it can be better for her than if the steward were always to show his true feelings.

If a nurse does not actually have caring feelings for a patient she might nevertheless care enough (according to senses **B** and **C**) to act as if she does.

## PELLEGRINO'S FOUR SENSES OF CARE

There are other accounts of care derived from analytic philosophy, though they are few and far between. For instance, Pellegrino (a male philosopher with an interest in medical ethics) also distinguishes four senses of care.[40]

The first is 'care as compassion' – feeling concerned for another person either by somehow sharing someone's experience of illness and pain, or just by being touched by their plight. The second sense is 'doing for others' what they cannot do for themselves – assisting with activities of daily living compromised by illness (feeding, bathing, clothing and so on). Pellegrino's third category is 'caring for the patient's medical problem', under which the carer invites the patient to transfer responsibility and anxiety about what is wrong to the doctor or nurse. His final sense is to 'take care', which means carrying out the necessary personal and technical procedures of care with conscientious attention.

Pellegrino's four senses can be summarised like this:

1. Caring by being concerned for another's welfare.
2. Caring by doing something for another's welfare.
3. Caring by taking on part of the burden of another's illness.
4. Caring by acting conscientiously.

For Pellegrino, these senses are inseparable in clinical practice. To perform them is to carry out 'integral care' which – in Pellegrino's opinion – is a moral obligation of health professionals.

There are similarities between Pellegrino's analysis of care and the **four types of caring** explained above (for example, his **4** and my **C**), but Pellegrino's moral commitment will not allow for pretence (so my **D** is not allowed on his scheme).

# CARING CONSTRUCTIVELY – DECIDING HOW TO CARE

As we have seen, because care is not a simple idea, theoretical and practical questions inevitably arise whenever a carer needs to decide which sort of care to offer. How is she to work out whether to become involved or to withdraw? How can she decide when to distance herself from her patient's worries, and when to hold his hand and cry with him? When should she put technical work before her personal feelings, and vice versa? Should she force herself to 'portray care' for a woman she dislikes? How can she distinguish appropriate caring activities from inappropriate ones?

Answers to these questions cannot be found in concepts of care alone (not even on Pellegrino's philosophical scheme, since his four senses do not of themselves explain why nurses ought to care integrally), nor can they be answered solely by intuition (feminine or masculine). They are possible only once **the point** of caring for specific people in specific situations has been established.

## A CLEAR PICTURE OF CARE

Care is a fairly complex idea, but it is not a primary nursing notion (see **Figure 3**).

Note that:

B can be done with or without **A**.
B can be done on its own, but is usually associated with **C**.
B can be done with **D**, and often is.
C can be done with or without **A**.
C can be done on its own, but is usually associated with **B** in practice.
C can be done with **D**, and often is.
D cannot be done with **A**.
A can be done without either **B**, **C** or **D**.

These last two are especially significant. Once appreciated they should remedy any over-enthusiasm for form **A** alone.

Though **D** (portraying care) cannot be combined with **A** (being emotionally involved), **D** can be beneficial in some situations, where it ought to be allowed to override **A**. But if **A** is considered to be what caring is all about, **D** is excluded.

Of course, form **A** is not necessarily detrimental on its own, but it can be. As everyone knows, emotional commitment can be volatile, unpredictable and upsetting.

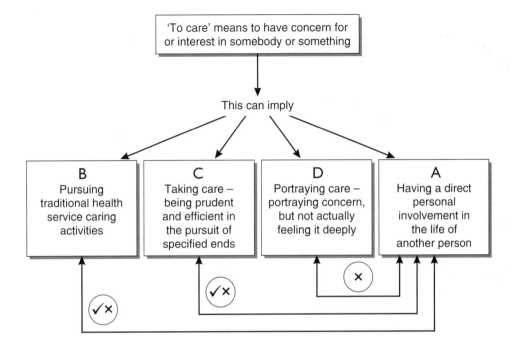

The carer constantly faces a fundamental question, namely:
Why should I choose A, B, C or D – or some combination?

However much she cares she is unable to decide unless she has a
governing theory – a theory beyond 'the ethics of care' – to help her do so

**Figure 3** Care defined and different forms of care distinguished

## THE IMPORTANCE OF EMOTION

None of this is to say that emotional involvement with patients is wrong, or that emotional involvement is not a central part of what caring means. Nor is it to say that nurses should be coldly analytical and switch their caring on and off at will.

Nursing is always an emotional experience and few of us can escape our emotions – nor ought we to try. If a nurse feels for a patient then she should accept it – she should perhaps even be grateful for it – unless her emotions become hazardous, or unless it becomes likely they will do more harm than good. At such a point the nurse ought to try to distance herself from her feelings or from the situation, and she should seek help if she cannot manage this alone.

This is no more manipulative than nurse theorists' encouragement to nurses to become fully involved in their patients' lives – to 'self-actualise' as they say. Like my proposal, their strategy asks that nurses work with and on their emotions – the difference is that the nurse theorists tell them to maximise rather than control their feelings.

The only alternative to not working either to control or develop one's emotions is to feel and act spontaneously on every occasion – but it does not take much imagination to picture the chaos this might cause.

The scheme I am proposing in this book (see **Chapters Nine** and **Ten** especially) urges emotional and moral commitment – but only so much of it as is good for the health of the nurse and the patient. It recognises that the most important of all nursing moments are precisely those times of intense feeling shared with patients: a sharing of brute reality, a privileged insight into the true depth of the human experience. But it also recognises that nursing has other ends too, and that these need to be balanced against rushes of emotion.

Too much or too little emotion can be crushing and nurses who want to work for health need a way to help them deal with it when they see either happening to them or to others.

# THE NEED FOR A GOVERNING THEORY TO DIRECT THE CARER

As can be seen from **Figure 3**, a carer needs to do more than care in order to decide which form of care to use in a particular situation. She must ask: why should I choose **A**, **B**, **C**, **D** or some combination? And she will be unable to answer her question unless she has a governing theory to help her.

There are many alternative governing theories she might choose. For the sake of illustration, briefly consider how two possible options – **Economic Rationalism** and **Caring as Giving Strength** – might function.

## USING ECONOMIC RATIONALISM AS A GOVERNING THEORY

Assuming that economic rationalism (**ER**) means:

> **Maximise the effectiveness of health services for the lowest possible financial cost**

it is easy to work out how **ER** would advise the carer who asks: **how should I care for this person in these circumstances?**

In every possible circumstance **ER directs that she should use that form of care most likely to bring about a technically and fiscally efficient outcome**. In practice this usually means that the carer should choose the least time-consuming form of care, the one which uses least resources and which produces a pre-specified service outcome to a set standard of effectiveness. For example, imagine a nurse asking: how ought I to care for Margaret, who is so terrified of an operation she is unable to sign the consent form? The **ER** governing theory must recommend that she use one or more of the forms **B**, **C** and **D** in order to 'consent' the patient at the earliest opportunity. The **ER** theory could not advise option **A** since this would mean that the nurse would have to

## ECONOMIC RATIONALISM
## AS A GOVERNING THEORY

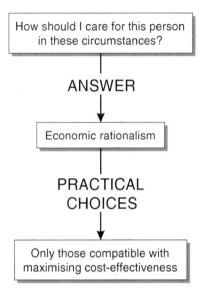

How should I care for this person
in these circumstances?

# ANSWER

Economic rationalism

# PRACTICAL
# CHOICES

Only those compatible with
maximising cost-effectiveness

**Figure 4**  Economic rationalism as a governing theory

strive to see the situation from the patient's point of view, empathise, counsel and probably educate as well (worthless goals in these circumstances, according to **ER**). It might even mean that the operation would be postponed, so incurring 'unnecessary' costs to the health system.

## USING CARING AS GIVING STRENGTH AS A GOVERNING THEORY

Assume that the basic idea of **caring as giving strength** is that:

> **The carer should select the type of care most likely to make the recipient physically, mentally, emotionally and spiritually stronger**

On this theory a nurse might ask: why is Margaret terrified? Is she adequately protected from undue pressure? Does she have enough information to reach a balanced judgement? Is she sufficiently educated to enable her to make a well-reasoned decision about how to proceed? Is she aware of other people who have been in this situation?

In this case – unlike **ER** – the **caring as giving strength** theory permits the use of option **A**. If it seems that option **A** will increase Margaret's strength to deal with this traumatic situation then the nurse can choose to use it. If not she will need to select an alternative type.

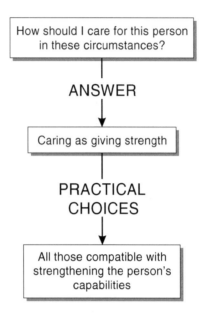

**Figure 5**    Giving strength as a governing theory

She might form a view that the operation will considerably enhance Margaret's physical strength in the long run, and then use some combination of boxes **B, C** and **D**. For instance, she might decide that time is of the essence, or she may discover that Margaret needs someone to take charge for her (perhaps the nurse finds out that Margaret has regular operations and always reacts like this, has the decision taken out of her hands, and is very grateful afterwards).

At some point, even on the **caring as giving strength** theory, the nurse might have to take account of economic considerations, but these would not be the ultimate guide to her thinking.

# CHAPTER FOUR

# Dignity

## SUMMARY

This chapter:

1. Explains why a practical understanding of dignity is needed.
2. Explains **two types** and **four levels** of dignity loss.
3. **Defines dignity**.
4. Provides an image of dignity that can help nurses promote dignity when it is lacking.

———————— ◆ ————————

---

*CASE THREE*

### Phoebe Undignified

Everyone agrees Phoebe is mentally competent. Every day she tells Ann that she wishes only to sit in her room – reading, thinking and watching the world pass by – and would like her meals there. She prefers to be alone and does not want to mingle with other old people.

However it is 'house policy' that everyone eats together. They must also vacate their rooms for several hours each day, unless they are ill.

Phoebe is normally able to decide what she eats, when she eats it and who she eats with. Now she cannot, and she feels bereft.

Most of the other staff think it obvious that patients should spend their days in the Day Room – what else is it for? Ann complains that it is undignified for Phoebe to be treated like this, but her objections are brushed aside. Her colleagues don't understand what she is talking about. 'Phoebe is a very dignified lady', 'It is only a few hours a day and she doesn't have to talk to people she doesn't want to', 'It isn't good for her to shut herself away like that', they say when challenged.

To those staff for whom 'upholding patient dignity' means anything, it means that residents should be decently dressed, bathe regularly and live as normal a life as possible,

*continues*

— *continued* —

with meals at set times and bed-time at 10.30 p.m. An orderly, conventional life must be a dignified one, they tacitly assume. Ann disagrees but struggles to articulate her dissent. She needs a way to spell out the constituents of dignity — she needs to be precise in order to demonstrate the indignity the residential unit's policy is causing Phoebe.

*SECTION ONE*

# THE NEED FOR DIGNITY

'Mission statements' and Codes of Practice regularly assert a commitment to patient dignity (see also **Chapter One**). Unfortunately, this worthy ideal often becomes lost beneath more tangible clinical and managerial priorities. When resources are scarce and there is a host of very visible technical problems to deal with, it is all too easy to neglect patient dignity.

## A PRESSING CONTEMPORARY PROBLEM

At the time of writing there is plentiful evidence that patients – particularly mentally vulnerable and elderly people – are not being treated with dignity.

A campaign entitled 'Dignity on the Ward' was initiated by the *Observer* newspaper in the UK in 1997 in response to complaints from relatives of older people about poor standards of care in the National Health Service. This prompted the then Health Secretary Frank Dobson to commission a study of 16 randomly selected acute wards in general hospitals. The subsequent report **'Not Because They are Old'**[41] showed that older patients and their relatives were less satisfied with care than other age groups. In particular:

> ...there were problems with preserving dignity and individuality when meeting patients' essential needs (personal hygiene, dressing). Some of these were related to the poor physical environment, but some were due to staff attitudes.[41]

It recommended:

> Better education and training... for staff about the specific needs of older people irrespective of where they work.[41]

The UK *Guardian* of 23 January 1999 carried the following story:

> A damning report yesterday on abuse at an NHS hospital revealed that nurses hit and tied up elderly mentally ill patients, and racially intimidated colleagues who threatened to report them.
> The 18-month inquiry found that the 13 residents of Beech House, a geriatric unit in St. Pancras Hospital, central London, were forced to bathe in freezing water, hit with shower heads, unnecessarily moved in the night and verbally bullied during the period from the unit's opening in March 1993 until its closure three years later.

A **Help the Aged** report published on 14 September 1999 claimed that old people in Britain are being forced to live in conditions similar to those found in Victorian Workhouses.

The report followed revelations that some residents are woken at 4.30 a.m. (a convenient time for staff) and forced to have tea. It was also discovered that others are made to sit in chairs for hours, even if they have medical conditions exacerbated by extended sitting.[42]

Help the Aged found that elderly people are not allowed to make decisions about their future and are often forced unnecessarily into residential homes, against their wishes. The report suggested that simple technology could be used to allow people to stay in their homes, yet it is not provided. Remote control door locks and window openers, lighting to illuminate the way to the bathroom at night and movement detectors to alert a response centre if a person does not get up in the morning could be all it takes to make the difference between independence and dependence.

The nursing literature shows that these problems are not new:

> Examples of the kind of control over patients exercised by the ward staff occurred principally when they were not being closely supervised by Sister Green . . . there was a tendency to issue peremptory commands and reprimands; for example – a patient who was attempting to drink undiluted orange squash from a bottle was shouted at to 'Stop that', but no glass of water was provided to enable him to have a drink . . .
> . . . a patient who was unable to speak was found by a SEN* to be resting on his bed after lunch, and told that this was not allowed and that he was to go back to the Day Room. He got up but, as soon as the SEN had gone, went back to his bed. The SEN returned and sent him to the Day Room but the same thing happened again. Finally, the SEN started to escort the patient to the Day Room, the patient looked harassed, the SEN appeared to be amused . . .
> Interrelated with their belief that the patients should be controlled was the importance the ward staff attached to 'getting through' [the work] and 'getting straight', i.e. achieving a tidy ward . . . The routine involved the unvarying performance of certain tasks in a pre-determined order which limited considerably the extent to which patients' individual requirements could be accommodated.[43] (*SEN means State Enrolled Nurse)

The great majority of health professionals want to uphold human dignity. The problem is that until dignity is recognised as a palpable concept, its provision is unlikely to be a practical priority.

Fortunately, it is possible to make dignity explicit, through philosophical analysis. The following section shows how.

*SECTION TWO*

# WHAT IS DIGNITY?

To read most Codes of Practice one might think 'dignity' requires no definition.

The Australian Nurses' Code of Ethics states:

> Respect for individual needs, beliefs and values includes culturally sensitive care, and the provision of as much comfort, dignity, privacy and alleviation of pain and anxiety as possible.[44]

The Nurses' Code of Conduct 1995 instructs each nurse to:

> ...respect the dignity, culture, values and beliefs of patients...[45]

And the Commonwealth Standards for Nursing Homes says:

> It is the responsibility of nursing home management to ensure that the privacy and dignity of residents are respected.[46]

The UK Patient's Charter states that patients can:

> ...expect the NHS to respect your privacy, dignity and religious and cultural beliefs at all times and in all places.[47]

And the United Kingdom Central Council for Nurses, Midwives and Health Visitors Code of Professional Conduct (1992) instructs that:

> ...in the exercise of your professional accountability, [you] must recognise and respect the uniqueness and dignity of each patient and client.[48]

In each case the nature of dignity is taken as read. But without a definition of dignity and a list of practical conditions that must be provided to ensure it, the aspiration to achieve it is toothless – particularly where finances are tight and an institution's culture firmly set.

## CHALLENGING QUESTIONS

In order to achieve a decisive account of dignity it is necessary to answer some challenging questions. These are:

1. **What are the constituents of dignity?**
2. **Are these constituents universally required?**
3. **Is dignity a matter of degree, or does one either have it or not?**
4. **How can nurses work practically to ensure their patients have dignity?**

# A PHILOSOPHICAL ANALYSIS OF DIGNITY

It is possible to discover the meaning of dignity by carefully examining situations in which we lack it or are at risk of losing it.

## LACK OF DIGNITY

What makes people feel undignified? Reflection on personal experience shows we tend to lack dignity when we find ourselves in inappropriate circumstances – when we are in situations where we feel foolish, incompetent, inadequate, or unusually vulnerable.

To spell this out a little more, we may lack dignity:

In circumstances ill-fitted to our competencies (Type 1)

and

In circumstances in which we are normally capable, but where we fail to achieve what we routinely would (Type 2)

We do not necessarily lack dignity under these conditions. And when we do experience indignities they are not always of the same magnitude.

## LEVELS OF DIGNITY LOSS

It is helpful to distinguish different levels of dignity loss. Like the two **types** above, these are not absolutely separate categories, but they do begin to offer a more complete picture of dignity:

 i. **Dignity maintained.**
 ii. **Dignity lost in a trivial way – dignity easily restored.**
 iii. **Serious loss of dignity – substantial effort and probably help from others required to restore it.**
 iv. **Devastating loss of dignity – impossible for a person to regain dignity without help.**

By combining these **levels** with the two general **types** we discover **eight kinds of situation in which dignity is either at risk or lost**.

**1i. A person is in circumstances ill-fitted to her competencies, but dignity is maintained**
Inappropriate circumstances are common in everyone's life, and always carry the risk of dignity loss. How we respond – or are able to respond – can make the difference between dignity maintained and dignity lost.

Peter is a high-flyer. He's not yet 30 and has progressed rapidly, specialising in urology. He has been courted by two large clinical departments who would both like him to accept a post as Senior Theatre Nurse with a view to management in a year or two. However, Peter has decided to become a nurse academic and has applied for a newly established Chair in Clinical Nursing at the local University.

He is a clever, hard-working nurse and has never failed to secure any job he's been interviewed for. The word is he will get the job, and leave his present position shortly.

His colleagues are in the middle of arranging a celebration bash (which they intend to keep secret just in case he is disappointed) when Peter walks in, looking downcast. He sees what they are doing and blushes deeply.

This is a new experience for him. For a moment he doesn't know what to do. He feels like crying and is in danger of losing his dignity.

Then four pagers go off at once. There is an emergency in theatre and they need Peter immediately.

Instantly he forgets his embarrassment, regains his composure, and dashes to the theatre to change.

Peter nearly lost his dignity because he was incompetent to deal with the circumstances he found himself in. Fortunately, the circumstances changed, ensuring that his dignity was maintained.

He has learnt from the experience (his capabilities have expanded as a result of it). If he ever finds himself in a similar situation he now knows that the adage 'win some lose some' applies to everyone – even him – and he backs himself to win more than he loses. 'Their loss, not mine', he'll say. He'll be hurt but he'll shrug it off and enjoy his friends.

Because he now has the capabilities to deal with such circumstances he will be able to maintain dignity if they ever occur again.

**2i. A person is in circumstances in which she is normally capable, fails to achieve what she routinely would, yet still maintains her dignity**
We can usually excuse ourselves if we find we have bitten off more than we can chew. But if we fail to do what we have come to take for granted, that can be harder to bear.

It is possible to maintain dignity in these circumstances, but the person in the risky situation must have other useful capacities and be able to draw on them. For example, at 72 Brian Smith had a stroke which resulted in a right-sided weakness which meant he was unable to walk unaided. Mr Smith previously had an active life and was captain of the local bowls team. For several weeks after his discharge from hospital he tried to carry on playing, and held onto the captaincy even though he was so frustrated at his reduced playing abilities that he couldn't concentrate on leadership.

No one told him to give it up, but he began to notice too many pitying, embarrassed looks in his direction. Brian dug deep. He tried to look at himself from the others' point of view. He didn't like what he saw, felt profoundly sorry for himself for an hour, and then volunteered to retire from playing and offered to assist with the administrative aspects of the bowls club instead (he used to be a senior bank official). His offer was accepted with delight and relief by the rest of the team.

Brian Smith had managed to maintain his dignity. He changed the prevailing circumstances as best he could. He was no longer able to play bowls properly but maintained his dignity because he had additional competencies which he could bring into play to improve his vulnerable situation.

(Thanks to Ann Gallagher for this example.)

**1ii. A person is in circumstances ill-fitted to his competencies and loses dignity in a trivial way**
Like **1i**, this is a common state of affairs. The over-confident driver who has to drive a vehicle with more power than he is used to, the childless woman who thinks mothering comes naturally and who offers to take on a group of three-year-olds for the morning, the student nurse who undertakes to remove a drain even though she has only ever practised on a model – each is at risk of at least a trivial loss of dignity.

I recently experienced this category. I am (or was) just about adequate at outdoor cricket, and had been invited to play indoor cricket for the first time. I was confident my skills would transfer to the indoor game readily enough, but unfortunately there are significant differences between the two versions. In indoor cricket the batting side has 5 runs deducted each time the batsman is out, but he or she bats on until four overs have been completed. The indoor court is small and surrounded by a taut net from which the ball rebounds to fielders if struck with any power. The idea is basically to 'tip and run'. The last thing the batsman should do is play standard cricket strokes – a truth painfully revealed to me in the space of 24 deliveries, during which I was out seven times (so scoring minus 35).

This was a relatively trivial indignity, and was annulled in part by self-deprecating humour and the promise to shout the drinks if it happened in the next match (assuming I would be asked to contribute to another game). I could avoid deeper indignity because I was able to find a strategy to laugh it off, because indoor cricket isn't important to me, and because there are quite a few things in life that I am good at.

### 2ii. A person is in circumstances in which she is normally capable, fails to achieve what she routinely would, and loses dignity in a trivial way
This combination is likely to be tougher to deal with than situations in which one has no previous expertise, but can be solved by a dignified strategy.

A nurse who fluffs some simple (non-dangerous) calculations whilst preparing medications may be embarrassed and lose some dignity, but if she can explain the lapse to others, and if she is generally capable, she will be able to avoid further indignity.

### 1iii. A person is in circumstances ill-fitted to her competencies, and suffers a serious loss of dignity
This state of affairs can occur when people are promoted beyond their abilities, for example. It also arises in various ways in hospitals and other health service settings. It can, for instance, be difficult for even the most scrupulous nurse to remember that her familiar work setting may seem alien to a newly admitted patient. Unless the patient is told the routines, knows where the toilets are, can find a telephone, and can have privacy when she needs it she may well suffer a serious loss of dignity. If she has good personal resources available – if she is cogent, if she can walk, if she has the confidence to speak out then she may be able to regain dignity herself. But if she does not possess these assets then she may even sink into category 1iv.

### 2iii. A person is in circumstances in which she is normally capable, fails to achieve what she routinely would, and suffers a serious loss of dignity
Such predicaments sometimes occur in health service institutions – especially those that are under-resourced. A few years ago in England a charge nurse called Graham Pink blew the whistle on just such a situation – a geriatric ward of 24 patients for whom he had to care single-handed every night he was on duty.[49] He told the world, via the *Guardian* newspaper, that he commonly had to leave intellectually competent elderly people on commodes for an hour or more, and that sometimes they had to sit in soiled bedclothes for as long.

The elderly people's dignity was undermined because the hospital was unable to ensure that they could do what they would normally take for granted – the hospital thus failed to provide for their dignity.

Phoebe (featured in **Case Three** at the head of this chapter) is in this category. She is normally capable of making routine meal-time choices, but is prevented from making these everyday decisions by the residential home's policies. This seems a trivial matter to some of the staff, but for Phoebe to lose this independence – to fail to achieve what she normally would in such mundane circumstances – is a serious loss of dignity.

### 1iv. A person is in circumstances ill-fitted to her competencies and suffers a devastating loss of dignity

A person newly diagnosed with a serious disease might find herself in this unhappy state of affairs. She may be at a complete loss about what to do and will require sensitive, practical support to liberate new or latent capabilities, and so regain dignity.

### 2iv. A person is in circumstances in which she is normally capable, fails to achieve what she routinely would, and suffers a devastating loss of dignity

Such a situation might happen following chemotherapy, for example. At visiting time a patient might be unable to speak with her gathered family because she is constantly vomiting. If so she may require urgent help from others to rediscover her dignity. Health workers must either rapidly change her circumstances or they must equip her with new competencies to ensure that she can cope with her indignity.

## GENERAL AND SPECIFIC DEFINITIONS OF DIGNITY

The above analysis suggests that **dignity always has to do with being in a position where one is capable**. When an elderly person in a rest home is placed in a room painted in a colour she hates, is given food she dislikes, is treated as unintelligent when she is bright, and is not allowed to choose what time she goes to bed, it is unlikely she will feel dignified, simply because she has not been allowed to be capable.

Dignity may be generally defined like this:

> **A person will have dignity if he is in a situation where his capabilities can be effectively applied**

Dignity may be defined more specifically like this:

> **This person's capabilities are A, B, C…X, Y, Z. She will have dignity in situations where she can exercise these capabilities effectively**

Other analysts have arrived at similar conclusions (welcome examples of nurse theorists undertaking analytic philosophy properly). Elaine Mairis asked 20 nursing students what dignity means. She concluded that:

> Dignity may be said to exist when an individual is capable of exerting control or choice over his or her behaviour, surroundings and the way in which he or she is treated by

others. He or she should be capable of understanding information and making decisions. He or she should feel comfortable with his or her psychosocial *status quo*.[50]

Jane Haddock considers that:

> Dignity is the ability to feel important and valuable in relation to others, communicate this to others, and be treated as such by others, in contexts which are perceived as threatening...possession of dignity within oneself affects one's ability to maintain or promote the dignity of another.[51]

Both writers have discovered that dignity depends upon a person's ability. And since ability is dependent on circumstances (it's no use being a wonderful ball-player if you don't have a ball) dignity promotion may best be summed up like this:

**If a health worker wants to promote a person's dignity she must either expand her capabilities or improve her circumstances**

Research and motivation are necessary in order to discover what any particular person's capabilities are. It is obviously wrong, for example, to assume that every elderly person has the same potential. For dignity's sake it is vital to match things provided to an individual's potential capability. Such methods as the 'Resident Categorisation Instrument'[52] may be one way to begin such an investigation, but more depth is needed genuinely to find out what dignity means for each person.

Occasionally a person will need only one capability – the mental strength to cope with not having any others. Indeed, there can be great dignity in dealing with profound or insuperable difficulty – such as the death of a loved one. In this case a person's capabilities are brought to bear on a problem with supreme appropriateness: I can't do this, I can't change that, but I can say this and I can carry on – this is how I am coping.

*SECTION THREE*

# PROMOTING DIGNITY

**Some Questions**

The above distinctions are not the whole story. Dignity is a rather elusive notion, and there are other questions to consider before it can be fully understood.

**Question 1: Are certain provisions or conditions necessary to the dignity of any human being?**
Yes, generally speaking. In order to be capable everyone needs certain resources. Just to carry out our daily tasks we usually need physical strength, freedom from debilitating thoughts and emotions, information, time, freedom from overwhelming life stresses, and so on. There are a few cases in which this set of conditions does not apply – they do not apply to the ascetic, the person who carries out a dignified suicide in order to escape an intolerable illness, or the person who will risk everything for a cause – but it is otherwise pervasive.

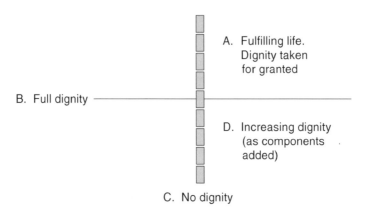

**Figure 6**   Dignity depicted

**Question 2: Does a person either have dignity or not, or is dignity a matter of degree?**
Both of these are possible. It could be that one event in category **1iv** or **2iv** – say losing one's job or being revealed as a fraud – is enough to strip a person of all dignity. However, it is also possible that though such traumas may reduce victims' capabilities dramatically, there may still be many aspects of their lives in which they remain capable – in which case they will be in categories **1iii** or **2iii** (and somewhere between **B** and **C** on **Figure 6**). In straitened circumstances it is often by means of doing certain other things well (holding the family together, searching intelligently and with commitment for new work, decorating the house, not going to pieces) that a person retains dignity.

## OFFERING PRACTICAL DIGNITY TO PHOEBE

Dignity seems to be constructed like a brick wall, made up of numerous capabilities of many different kinds, assembled as the years go by.

This suggests an interesting – and practically helpful – image (see **Figure 6**).

Most people living regular lives at study, in employment, or in productive retirement are at **A**. We are fortunate in having dignity because we are in situations appropriate to our capabilities. Indeed, most of us would have full dignity even if we lost some of our capacities.

Because we are in such good positions there is usually considerable leeway between losing our options and losing our dignity altogether. A person might lose her possessions in a flood, her car in an accident, and her husband to another woman and retain a degree of dignity because she still has other resources on which to call. She might retain pride, belief in herself, her job and so be able to set about rebuilding her wall of dignity back up to **B**: the threshold for full dignity.

Of course, people at position **A** might still lose dignity, from time to time, in the less serious ways, but will quickly be able to regain it. The inept sporting performance, the

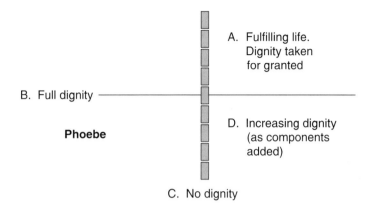

**Figure 7**   Phoebe's dignity depicted

ungainly fall, the idiotic comment in conversation, a lack of discretion brought on by alcohol – all these are quickly recoverable.

Elderly people are less likely than most to be at **A**. When caring for elderly people the health worker who wishes to enhance dignity should try to find out what the person in question has been capable of, what he is capable of now, and what his priorities are. The health worker should also try to provide the wherewithal to permit the person to achieve his goals. As a priority she should create situations which promote his capabilities up to point **B**. The worker should also seek to prevent situations in which his patients might feel foolish and incompetent. For example, a nurse who wants to uphold the dignity of her Alzheimer's patient might engage him in conversation on a topic he judges important (a respected colleague of mine once nursed a patient who enjoyed discussing Aussie rules football, and another who was an authority on dogs). By doing this, boredom and frustration are eliminated and the patient's capabilities are both respected and reinforced. This is a specific way to foster dignity – and does not depend on woolly sentiment.

## CREATING DIGNITY IS WORK FOR HEALTH

Phoebe is here on this image (see **Figure 7**).

In order to promote dignity the very first priority is to get her to line **B**. Her health workers should then strive to keep her there and so give her the opportunity to live in the ways of her choosing – she should be at **B** so she can continue to carve out a fulfilling life for herself.

Either those in charge of Phoebe's institution wish to promote dignity or they do not. If they do, then – since Phoebe's ability to decide for herself is essentially undiminished – they **must** change Phoebe's circumstances because their inflexible rules are damaging her dignity. They must let her eat where she likes.

**Question 3: Are there circumstances and goals beyond dignity? Is there a point at which a person can be said to have dignity to which improved circumstances could not add?**

If **Figure 6** is correct then the answer to this question is clearly yes. If one is at **B** or above then dignity is not an issue – one has capabilities suited for all the circumstances one normally finds oneself in. If, for instance, you have money, work, a home, friends, confidence and optimism then you will have full dignity – it will never occur to you that your dignity might be threatened.

**Question 4: Is dignity entirely to do with how a subject feels? Can a person be undignified even if he feels dignified, or if he doesn't realise he is undignified?**

This is a philosophically interesting question, though not central to the current discussion. However it may be worth saying a little about it.

Dignity must be sensed – to feel dignity or not is an experience. Consider a case in which a person under anaesthetic is left naked on an operating table in public view – but never knows it. At first sight it seems natural to say that the person suffered an indignity – but in truth he or she did not suffer anything. Only if he finds out what happened could he possibly feel undignified.

There is indignity here, but it is experienced vicariously. The doctor or nurse who finds the patient unnecessarily exposed will likely think either that Mr X would not wish to be seen like this, I would not wish to be seen like this, or most people would not wish to be seen like this. Strictly speaking, in such cases we rightly apply a generally held understanding of dignity to prevent what would be indignities, were they actually experienced by the subject. Our own sense of dignity is protected as we act in what we assume to be another person's interests, when he cannot act for himself.

In the case of a person who looks undignified to an observer but does not think he lacks dignity, so long as he understands what dignity means then he cannot be undignified, whatever the onlooker thinks. The person who genuflects in front of a monarch can – in some people's eyes – appear undignified, though he may see his behaviour as the height of dignity. To give another illustration, the smelly vagrant dressed in rags begging in the street seems undignified to most of us – but she may very well not see her situation like this. She may be surviving as best she can, and this may give her a great sense of dignity.

Of course she may indeed feel that she lacks dignity. And if we care about what happens to her then we will find out what she thinks, and help her if we can.

**Question 5: Does a person have to be observed to feel undignified?**

Though a person obviously does not have to be directly and constantly seen by others to lack dignity, witnessing is still an important notion. As far as trivial indignities are concerned, being observed can make all the difference (if no one had been watching my hopeless display of indoor cricket I would not have felt I was losing my dignity, though I would have been annoyed with myself).

The more serious indignities (losing a job, losing a wife to an affair) tend to be made much worse because they are seen – or because of how we think we will be regarded by others. And if an indignity is entirely hidden from others it is made an indignity by the subject's own observation.

## CONCLUSION

By putting flesh on dignity's bones nurses are enabled to recognise clearly and immediately when dignity is missing (so long as they know what a patient's capabilities are). Because of this practical grounding, when a nurse says 'I believe in patient dignity' she will understand she is making a powerful, thoughtful and practical commitment to the welfare of others.

Dignity is important for its own sake, but it is even more important for what it allows a person to go on and do. This is the real reason for promoting dignity. It allows us to think positively of dignifying someone – even someone with very few potentials left open to him. When we understand dignity in this way we understand the importance of reflecting on human capabilities, and we know that if we have real concern for others we must do our utmost to find circumstances in which these capabilities can flourish.

(With thanks to Leila Shotton, who co-authored the earlier paper on which this chapter is based.)

# CHAPTER FIVE

# Holism and Separatism

## SUMMARY

This chapter:

1. Identifies two senses of holism – **strict** and **practical**.
2. Explains that holism can be a general inspiration for nursing.
3. Describes the contradiction between holism and nurse separatism.
4. Establishes that because nursing is a holistic enterprise, nurses cannot logically argue that they are separate from other health workers.
5. Suggests that because nursing is holistically inspired, nurses might take the lead in establishing a morally purposive health system.

———————— ◆ ————————

*SECTION ONE*

## HOLISM

Nurse theorists espouse holism almost as much as they praise advocacy, care and dignity. Time and again one reads that if nurses are to offer a viable alternative to reductionist medicine, they should practise holistically. But what does this mean?

## HOLISM'S SENSES

Holism is the idea that the whole is greater than the sum of the parts. It can be understood **strictly** or **practically**.

### STRICT HOLISM

**Strict holism** makes two claims.

**1. A whole cannot be fully understood even if all its parts are understood separately**
For example, a family might be dissected into smaller and smaller parts: father,

mother, son, daughter; male bodies and female bodies; physical condition of bodies; blood pressure of each body at time X, and so on. But however many divisions are made – physical, sociological, historical or whatever – according to **strict holism** even knowing them all would not be sufficient to understand the family as a whole. The non-specific emotions generated by the relationships between the family members, what it means to all of them to be together or apart, a continuing and historical sense of belonging or dissonance – all these things and more exist because the family exists, but they do not occur on any inventory of the smaller parts that make the family up. Dissect a family into its bits and something essential disappears.

Here is a second example: as we breathe in, odour molecules float into our noses and through the nasal cavities behind. If we want to smell a rose we sniff at it. The sniff causes the air to swirl around in the nasal cavity and brings the odour molecules into contact with two patches of hairy cells – the olfactory epithelia. When certain odour molecules land on the cell's hairs, the cells generate nerve signals. These signals pass up to a clump of nerves just above – the olfactory bulb – where they are partly classified. Then they continue along the olfactory nerve to the olfactory (smell) centre in the brain.[53]

But though correct on its own terms, this description fails to capture the importance of the experience of smelling a gorgeous rose on a sublime summer's evening.

**2. The separate parts of something cannot be fully understood apart from the whole**
**Strict holism** also holds that the parts of something cannot be adequately understood in isolation from the whole (for example, the son cannot be fully understood if you do not also know the family of which he is a part).

Strictly speaking, the reductionist approach on which most clinical care is based is incompatible with holism. For example, some psychiatrists argue that pharmacological therapies are an adjunct to other mental health work: they aren't the whole answer, but they do help. However, according to **strict holism**, offering a drug to deal only with a person's emotional problems will be counter-productive because it will act to obscure the real nature of her problem (which can be properly comprehended only by looking at her life as a whole).

It is impossible to nurse according to **strict holism** in modern health systems, since the implication is that nurses should not analyse situations, and should not use even those methods of reductionist medicine known to help patients (and nor should they employ analytic philosophy).[54]

## HOLONS

Fortunately, nurses inclined to holistic practice need not abandon the good that can come from understanding parts of things. Not only is it obviously helpful to open up a broken machine to see which bits need replacing, but the distinction between 'wholes' and 'parts' (on which **strict holism** relies) is flawed:

...what exactly do we mean by the familiar words 'part' and 'whole'? 'Part' conveys the meaning of something fragmentary and incomplete, which by itself has no claim to autonomous existence. On the other hand, a 'whole' is considered as something complete in itself which needs no further explanation. However, contrary to these deeply ingrained habits of thought and their reflection in some philosophical schools, 'parts' and 'wholes' in an absolute sense do not exist anywhere, either in the domain of living organisms, or in social organizations, or in the universe at large.

A living organism is not an aggregation of elementary parts, and its activities cannot be reduced to elementary 'atoms of behaviour' forming a chain of conditioned responses. In its bodily aspects, the organism is a whole consisting of 'sub-wholes', such as the circulatory system, digestive system, etc., which in turn branch into sub-wholes of a lower order, such as organs and tissues – and so down to individual cells, and to the organelles inside the cells. In other words, the structure and behaviour of an organism cannot be explained by, or 'reduced to', elementary physico-chemical processes; it is a multi-levelled, stratified hierarchy of sub-wholes, which can be conveniently diagrammed as a pyramid or an inverted tree...

The point first to be emphasized is that each member of this hierarchy, on whatever level, is a sub-whole or 'holon' in its own right – a stable, integrated structure, equipped with self-regulatory devices and enjoying a considerable degree of *autonomy* or self-government. Cells, muscles, nerves, organs, all have their intrinsic rhythms and patterns of activity, often manifested spontaneously without external stimulation; they are subordinated as *parts* to the higher centres in the hierarchy, but at the same time function as quasi-autonomous *wholes*. They are Janus-faced. The face turned upward, toward the higher levels, is that of a dependent part; the face turned downward, towards its own constituents, is that of a whole of remarkable self-sufficiency.[55]

Once it is recognised that there is never an absolute distinction between any 'whole' and any 'part' then **strict holism** collapses, and nurses can practise holistically – so long as they define what is meant by a 'whole' and a 'part' (the various holons) in each nursing situation.

## PRACTICAL HOLISM

What matters is that the nurse direct her work toward the care of the whole she defines. For instance, dependent on circumstances, the whole may be the disease, the patient, the family of which the patient is a part, a ward or a wider community. Whatever the case, what is practically important for holistic nursing is that the nurse must always be aware that whatever she does to the part-wholes (holons) not only has a specific effect on those part-wholes, but impacts both on the holons above and the holons below in the system. If she gives drugs to control infection, if she speaks privately to a wife about her husband's illness, if she brings an extra bed into the ward, or if she appoints a new employee she must recognise that by so doing she is not just altering a portion, she is affecting a range of associated holons. A person suffers an infection, the wife is part of a family, there are other people in the ward, and a new appointment doesn't just add a new body to the team – it alters the entire team.

There is no doubt that holistic practice can be a civilising contribution to medical and nursing care. However, for one reason or another health professionals (nurses included) sometimes forget the wider picture – perhaps it is too complex, too emotionally demanding, too hard to alter – whatever the case the fact remains that it is too often neglected. Simply by championing this elementary form of holism – and by practising according to it wherever possible – nurses can render health care more humane.

Even so, holism on its own is not enough to guide nursing practice specifically. All **practical holism** says is:

> Notice that there is more to your nursing than meets the eye – notice there is more to this infection than breeding bacteria, notice there is more to this wound than isolated pain, notice there is more to this pain than can be measured scientifically, notice there is more to this person than you can ever know. Notice these things and act accordingly as you carry out your tasks and offer your caring skills.

How and to what specific ends the nurse should provide his skills are matters the dictum 'practise holistically' does not address. Holism is a general reminder to think broadly, deeply, and as a consequence, kindly. But it is no more than this.

## SECTION TWO

## SEPARATISM

Some nurses insist nursing is separate from other disciplines in every possible way – practically, professionally, conceptually and ethically. The following remark typifies their point of view:

> Nursing is a separate discipline from the other professions involved in health care, and therefore we bring our own issues, concerns, problems and dilemmas into a health care arena in which we as nurses need to look for and work out a resolution.[56]

However, though it is true that there are 'issues, concerns, problems and dilemmas' specific to nursing, nurses also share countless concerns and tasks with other professions:

> ... in recent years the role of nurses has changed greatly, and specialised nurses such as clinical nurse consultants are now taking on roles that were previously the domain of doctors and other health professionals; and many of the roles that were once exclusively the domain of nurses are now being taken over by other health workers. For example, in many coronary care wards, nurses may take blood, insert cannulas, diagnose arrythmias and initiate emergency treatment – all actions that were previously taken by doctors. However, in the same areas, bed making may now be done by special bedmakers, chest physiotherapy will be given by physiotherapists, and all aspects of diet will be looked after by dietitians – all roles that were formerly performed by nurses. Indeed, many of the traditional role boundaries between the professions seem now to be defined more by customs or institutions than by specialised training or professional aptitude.[57]

Furthermore:

> ... 'some half of the younger doctors, in Britain at least, are women.'[58] There are also ... many men who choose to work in nursing ... many doctors choose to work

in ... palliative care (what might be considered a high-care area) and many nurses choose to work ... in intensive care units (a high-tech area) ...[59]

As a matter of fact the boundaries between nurse and non-nurse – and between women and men health carers – are evolving, permeable and constantly breached.

## HOLISM AND SEPARATISM – A REVEALING CONTRADICTION

It is enlightening to think about holism and separatism, not merely because they are among nursing's most discussed **big ideas**, but because reflecting on them offers an insight into the theoretical knot in which some nurse theorists have bound themselves (and their colleagues).

If it can be taken as read that all nurse theorists are in favour of holism in one form or another (and as far as I know there are no papers by nurse academics against holism) then those nurse theorists who also favour separatism hold a contradictory position.

The problem is surely obvious. According to many nurse theorists, nurses are meant to 'advocate' patients' fundamental needs, to care personally – even to the extent of understanding what life means to the patient – and to practise holistically – spurning false distinctions between symptom and patient, patient and the patient's life, and patients' lives and the social world. Yet at the same time nursing is meant to be a separate profession, treading a unique path as it tackles its own special issues.

Of course, these aspirations are oil and water. To care holistically nurses must understand their patients as physical, emotional, social and spiritual wholes. And they must also – necessarily – see their work as part of rather than separate from the broader enterprise of working for health. The patient is a holon (partly dependent on the nurse, but also partly in charge of all manner of sub-systems), the nurse is a holon, her medical colleagues are holons and the system in which they work (and on which they are all largely dependent) is a holon too.

To illustrate:

---

## CASE FOUR

### Donald

Donald is in the terminal stages of multiple sclerosis. He lies vanquished in a hospital ward specially designed to cater for the needs of young, dying patients (Donald is 46). It is an improbably pleasant place, sprawled on a sunny hill overlooking a green park, away from the rest of the hospital (and the rest of the world).

*continues*

*— continued —*

Donald shares his room with one other patient called Bruce, a few years his junior and also dying from a neurological disorder.

Donald has several physical problems. He is virtually paralysed, his body is horribly emaciated (naked he looks like a prisoner of war – which in a way he is), his sight is failing and he has uncomfortable, sickly-smelling pressure sores.

Today Bruce died, suddenly. Donald's devoted wife and his son (a frightened 19-year-old, finding it impossible to mature because of all the suffering he's seen his Dad undergo for the last 16 goddam years) are about to arrive for a visit.

◆

## POSSIBLE TASKS FOR THE SEPARATIST NURSE

If she believes that:

> Nursing is a separate discipline from the other professions involved in health care, and ... bring[s] [its] own issues, concerns, problems and dilemmas into a health care arena ...[56]

the separatist nurse must identify those features of Donald's case that are uniquely nursing's and deal with them in nursing's own way. This inevitably means she must break the 'whole situation' down into certain components.

In Donald's case the separatist nurse might identify these tasks as nursing's own:

- Pressure area care
- Treatment of the existing sores
- Monitoring and delivery of medications
- Monitoring physical signs
- Offering emotional support
- Talking with and listening to Donald
- Talking with and listening to Donald's family

It may be that there are special nursing concerns here – perhaps the nurse disagrees with the strength of a prescription, perhaps it is the nurse to whom Donald turns first for comfort, perhaps the nurse has a different view from the doctor about what to say to the family. However, it is very hard to see how any nurse can coherently maintain that these aspects ought to be dealt with separately, by a separate profession. Doctors, other health professionals and social workers (and anyone else who wants to care constructively for Donald) surely have an important part to play in Donald's care, the above list included.

## POSSIBLE TASKS FOR THE HOLISTIC NURSE

Different collections of health workers are bound to have some unique concerns. But what matters to patients is that whoever is caring for them is aware of the bigger picture. Donald has many problems, some of which **could** be dealt with separately (his sores could be treated without a word being said, for example). However, not to see Donald's situation in a potentially unbounded holistic way is surely to fail to see the full reality of his health problems.

The real picture (following Koestler) is potentially unbounded because all holons are linked in a complicated chain of other holons. It is up to the holistic health worker to identify the particular combination of holons most relevant in any given situation.

In this case, the practical holistic tasks for the nurse (or anyone else willing and able to work for Donald's health) are:

- Pressure area care
- Treatment of the existing sores
- Monitoring and delivery of medications
- Monitoring physical signs
- Offering emotional support
- Talking with and listening to Donald
- Talking with and listening to Donald's family
- Talking with and listening to other health workers to explain what the nurse knows of the broader picture, and to learn what others know
- With Donald and other health workers, deciding on and if necessary revising a plan designed to give Donald maximum possible dignity
- With Donald and other health workers, deciding on and continually revising a plan designed to bolster Donald's health

Most of these tasks are the same as the separatist ones, but they make sense only if they are seen as part of a wider picture – indeed they make full sense only if one asks the defining holistic question: **what is the point of doing any or all of these separate tasks?**

It is counter-productive to set nursing up as a separate discipline. Nurse theorists can be either separatist or holist, but they can't be both. If they are separatist then they need to say what it is that nurses can do that no other discipline can (and no nurse theorist has ever come up with such a thing). And if they are holist they must explicitly eschew separatism and proclaim nursing a **bonding discipline**.

## SEPARATISM IS DESTRUCTIVE

First, if everything about Donald is dissected into separate tasks to be done by separate professionals it is likely there will be misunderstanding, miscommunication and missed chances to improve Donald's life. Second, if nursing continues to try to distance itself from other health workers, who is there left to pull things together? If nursing truly has its 'own issues, concerns, problems and dilemmas', then who will bother to teach other health workers about the importance of caring, moral commitment, standing up for patients, and what true dignity is? Who will support junior doctors when they are belittled by their seniors? Who will counsel non-nurse managers who think they must put money ahead of everything else? Who will paint the broad picture when utilitarian-minded professionals decide that very old or very sick people should not be treated?

Who will do these things? It won't be separatist nurses because as soon as they say all professions have different priorities they **deny** holism in health care, and throw away the possibility of leading the system toward better ways.

The desire to be separate – to be one of us rather than one of them – is a universal human tendency. Yet it is an awful addiction that those who favour holism must fight against. Koestler explains it astutely:

> From the dawn of recorded history, human societies have always been fairly successful in restraining the *self-assertive* tendencies of the individual – until the howling little savage in its cot became transformed into a more or less law-abiding and civilized member of society. The same historical record testifies to mankind's tragic inability to induce a parallel sublimation of the *integrative tendency*. Yet . . . both the glory and the pathology of the human condition derive from our powers of self-transcendence, which are equally capable of turning us into artists, saints or killers, but more likely into killers. Only a small minority is capable of canalizing the self-transcending urges into creative channels. For the vast majority, throughout history, the only fulfilment of its need to belong, its craving for communion, was identification with clan, tribe, nation, Church, or party, submission to its leader, worship of its symbols, and uncritical, child-like acceptance of its emotionally saturated system of beliefs . . .
>     To put it in the simplest way: the individual who indulges in an excess of aggressive self-assertion incurs the penalties of society – he outlaws himself, he contracts *out* of the hierarchy. The true believer, on the other hand, becomes more closely knit *into it*; he enters the womb of his Church or party, or whatever social holon to which he surrenders his identity. For the process of identification in its cruder forms always entails, as we have seen, a certain impairment of individuality, an abdication of the critical faculties and of personal responsibility.[55]
>
> . . . it is the integrative tendency acting as a vehicle or catalyst which induces the change in morality, the abrogation of personal responsibility, the replacement of the individual's code of behaviour by the code of the 'higher component' in the hierarchy. In the course of this fatal process, the individual becomes to a certain extent de-personalized; he no longer functions as an autonomous holon or part-whole, but merely as a part. Janus no longer has two faces – only one is left, looking upward in holy rapture or in a moronic daze.[55]

This is not mere speculation. Nor is it exaggerated. Not only is there devastating evidence of the **integrative tendency** all around us, but it can be demonstrated by the simplest of experiments:

> Parties of schoolboys aged 14 to 15 were subjected to a quick – and bogus – psychological test; then each boy was told that he was either a 'Julius person' or an 'Augustus person'. No explanation was given of the characteristics of the Julius or Augustus people, nor did the boys know who the other members of their group were. Nevertheless, they promptly identified with their fictitious group, proud to be a Julius person or an Augustus person to such an extent that they were willing to make financial sacrifices to benefit their anonymous group brothers, and to cause discomfort to the other camp.[55]

## NURSING'S SEPARATIST TRAP

Nursing is presently trapped by both **self-assertion** and the **integrative tendency**.

Nursing is seeking independence (many nurses are exhibiting collective **self-assertion** as 'Julius people' rather than 'Augustus people'), but it also wants to practise holistically (even though this is an out and out contradiction).

Furthermore, nursing's strong **integrative tendency** is impairing countless nurses' critical faculties – for instance, to be a nurse theorist not only do you have to be a nurse, you have to be part of the nurse theorist club. Dissent (too much **self-assertion** as an independent-minded individual) even from the most blatant nonsense leads to isolation, perhaps even ostracisation. So most don't do it – it is better to be part of the supposed 'nursing whole', even at the cost of intellectual autonomy.

Look again at Watson's words (quoted in **Chapter Three**) and you see nursing running around in caged circles, not realising how trapped it has become:

> Noddings links caring to the feminine spirit, the eros, as contrasted with the masculine spirit, the logos. Gadow, myself and others posit caring as a moral ideal that guides and directs human actions, not just as a means, but a human end in and of itself that is of intrinsic value to human civilization. A critical point is that these values and views of woman and caring are not just woman values, but values for all humanity.[34]

Here is the **integrative tendency** – the undemonstrable assumption that there are feminine and masculine spirits, and they are separate:

> Nursing is feminine. It has woman values. Too much of the world is run according to masculine values. But the patriarchy has failed. So nursing must break away from male logic and care with 'inner love, peace and joy'. Our tribe has the answer – trust us, join us.

But then there is also the **belief in holism**:

> Woman values are (or should be) everyone's values. If we can sustain a caring world then this will benefit humanity as a whole. Our values have the answer for the rest of you too.

And Watson is partly right. Nursing does have values that can benefit everyone, as **Part Two** of this book demonstrates. But she is also partly wrong. Nursing is not a separate endeavour – at most it is a small holon in an indefinitely larger whole.

What is the way forward? Nursing must transcend the **integrative tendency**. It must have the courage to say:

> **Full independence is an illusion. To pursue it is madness. So we do not want full independence.**

Given the power of the **integrative tendency**, it is far from certain that any group of people has the strength to do such a courageous thing (for to do so they must forsake an 'emotionally saturated system of beliefs' – they must disown a comfortingly vague place they all call home). But nurses have plentiful other homes already (religions, political parties, families, localities, nations and so forth). And if any group of people can overcome the **integrative tendency** nurses can: because the logic of their values is to transcend the 'group mind' to pursue humane goals for everyone, and because they have continual, direct experience of the commonality of human need.

To overcome the **integrative tendency** nursing must foster **self-assertive** tendencies in its members, not so that they become dominant or gain unique territory to defend, but so that nurses can develop and apply their critical faculties to the systems in which they work, in order to make nursing's holistic values a practical reality.

To achieve this nurses need first to explain (or at least understand) these values more clearly. And they need then to work out ways to apply them to cause the rigid social holon we call 'health services' to metamorphose into a system where moral ends are held to be at least as important as technical ones.[15]

If they succeed, nurses could yet forge a unique role for themselves without having to assert their separateness. Nurses could establish a special place as a **caring, bonding holon** – as pioneers of a morally purposive health system.

# PART TWO

# How Nursing Could Take the Moral Lead in Health Care

# CHAPTER SIX

# Research

## SUMMARY

This chapter:

1. Examines research in its most basic form in order to show that we are all researchers.
2. Demonstrates that assumptions both **enable** and **restrict** research.
3. Points out the danger of allowing research questions to dictate research goals.
4. Urges nurses explicitly and routinely to research in accord with **the values of nursing**.
5. Offers the **Honest Researcher Test** to help them do so.
6. Sketches out possible research projects based on **caring theory**.

---

◆

---

## INTRODUCTION

This chapter has four sections. By means of a short tale about a prehistoric researcher, **Section One** shows how much and how routinely we each research in order to solve our daily problems. It also highlights the importance of observation, theory and hypothesis in empirical research. **Section Two** shows how values affect research. **Section Three** presents the **Honest Researcher Test**. **Section Four** describes what an explicitly value-based approach to nursing research would look like, and outlines what it might achieve.

## WHAT THE CHAPTER IS NOT ABOUT

This chapter is not about how to do nursing research. Many books already explain this well.[60-65] Readers should turn to these, or to the many other 'how to research' books available, for advice on method.

## PRIMAL RESEARCH

*I*

Mungda had been abandoned by her tribe. She had no idea why. All she knew was that she had woken and they had vanished. They had left her nothing — no weapons, no tools, no food. She had only her animal skin and some old straw and leaves in an empty, dripping cavern.

Mungda was angry, anxious, perplexed and sad, though she had no words for these feelings. She sat by the paling embers of last night's fire, looking out, waiting for the sky to lighten.

Starry black slid to deepest blue, then the edge flushed orange. After that the blue got less and less and in the end turned grey.

Shaking, she ran outside in the soft light, crying out after them. But there was nothing apart from the scrubby hillside and the forest below and the deafening birdsong suffocating her scream.

They had gone. They would not be back, she knew. She was all there was, and she felt sick and dizzy with it. Then she felt so hungry nothing else mattered.

It was the beginning of the cool season. There had been meat last night, but that had disappeared along with everything else. All the local food — berries, roots and the like — had been exhausted by the tribe. And she had nothing to kill with. What was Mungda to do?

◆

### MUNGDA THE RESEARCHER

Though Mungda lived in a bygone world, we might still learn from her. She had no laboratory, no degrees, and no status, but she was as intelligent and inventive as we are. In fact Mungda was as good a researcher as most of those who work with today's sophisticated concepts.

This may seem a strange idea. An unkempt prehistoric woman, with barely any language, within a day or two of a wretched death, is not the conventional picture of a researcher. We are accustomed to thinking of research as a refined, intellectual activity. But at bottom it is nothing other than a purposeful examination of things we can experience.

If Mungda is to survive she has to explore her world in order to find an answer to her immediate problem. Unless she just happens across something to eat, she will have to do some research – she will have to observe, assess evidence, ask questions, come up with answers, devise theories and work out what will happen if she acts.

---

*II*

There was nothing in the cave for her. No point going back there, unless she needed shelter. But it wasn't yet so cold that she wanted to bury herself, and there was no evidence of fierce animals. So where should she go?

She noticed a rock steaming slightly against the pastel sun, and sat hunched up on it to think. The forest was below, perhaps with food eventually, but no guarantee of it and any number of unknown dangers hidden there. Above the cave the ground was rocky and steep, and behind the mountain ridge was the dry plain she had crossed with the others.

All she could see from the rock was forest. But she remembered it wasn't just forest down there. Coming over the mountain she had seen beyond the bush, to other hills. She needed to know more, so she needed to see more, and so she needed to climb back up the mountain. If she was going to die at least she would not do it as a dumb, abandoned animal.

---

◆

---

## BASIC RESEARCH

Mungda is facing the most basic problem of life – where can I find food? She has no knowledge of modern research techniques, yet she is a researcher because she is deliberately investigating both her inner world and the world beyond in order to solve a problem.

She is not aware she has theories, to her they are simply part of what she is. But she does have them. They are her interpretation of the world, derived from countless observations of what happens around her, to her and within her.

Her theories include: the knowledge that she needs to eat to carry on living (based on instinct and observation of people starving during periods of famine), the belief that dangers and opportunities will be more or less the same in the future as they were in the past (an opinion based on all her life's observations), the belief that observing as much as possible will give her a greater chance of solving her problem, and the belief that if she anticipates what might happen she stands a better chance than if she reacts instinctively (a view based on observation of the failures of impetuous tribesmen).

Not all her theories are testable. Some of them – like her sense that the sun is a god and should be worshipped, and that her ancestors watch over her – are matters of faith. But many of her understandings can be – and continually are – checked against the world.

## III

Turning her back on the warming sun, hotly angry and determined to live, Mungda began to climb.

Everything was alive for her. The green smell of the morning forest swam up to her, then sank into the red dust that rose as she walked. The birds were quieter as the sun climbed and she left them behind, but there were rustles and cracks and rattles everywhere. The mountain was bristling with life. She could hear its blood pulsing as it ran down to the wood.

She bent to put her hand in it. It bubbled over her palm and the mound of her thumb, glistening round and sparkly as it spurted over and on down the hill. She caught it and drank, and then some more. She was so dry, but the chilled mountain stream snatched her thirst away. She strode on, reaching the summit before the sun had got even half way into the sky.

Mungda turned, and looked. Not desperately, but with purpose. Where would there be food? And past that, where would there be safety? And beyond that, where could she rest and think some more?

She looked over her shoulder, to check that they were not on the plain. Then she looked at the forest spread out below her, and the hills blue green far away – too far for her ever to get to. It was as she'd remembered. But it wouldn't speak to her. She would have to force it to tell her where the food was. What could she see that could help her?

She looked down, her attention caught by the flash of the water growing as it got lower. That was there if she got thirsty again. But where did it go? As it entered the wooded area the water disappeared. It must have gone underground. Where else could it be?

She wished it would not disappear because lower down it would have to go somewhere and eventually there would be more of it, and there might be food for her in it. Perhaps it does come out, she thought. And so she began to look for it. And – because she was looking for water and not just at the forest as a whole – she saw that it did come out, though only to vanish again into the deep bush. If she found it and followed it she might yet be saved.

## RESEARCH IN ACTION

Mungda is making important steps in her research. She has observed, applied theories to her observations, and in the process has come up with a new theory. And not only this – now she has a hypothesis to test.

Here's some of her thinking so far:

1. Everything falls to earth eventually so this water will flow downhill until it can't go any further.
   **A theory based on countless observations.**

2. Either the water goes underground and stays there or it forms a pool in the forest.
   **A guess (or hypothesis) based on theory and observation.**

3. The water seems to go underground and emerge again – there will be a pool.
   **Another hypothesis.**

4. Big areas of water contain things I can eat.
   **A theory based on past observations and experiments and never yet shown to be wrong, in Mungda's experience.**

5. If I follow the path of the water I will find something to eat.
   **This is a further guess – a bolder hypothesis. But it is a potentially useful guess because Mungda will be able to experiment to see if it is correct.**

6. I must go down the mountain, follow the water and try to find food where the water stops.
   **Mungda concludes that she must carry out more research. If she succeeds she will gain knowledge as well as food.**

---

*IV*

The sun was ahead of her now. She knew it wouldn't get much higher and that she would need it in the forest. So she began to scurry and slide through the rocks and scree.

Though she was feeling light with hunger her outrage grounded her and made sure she didn't fall, and soon she was past the deserted cave without a glance. She followed the water, her feet breaking brown grass while the stream fizzed as it gathered pace.

The sun was past its climax as she entered the bush, but she could see well because she was not yet beneath the foliage. But soon the trees were taller, their branches cast shadows on her face and she hoped they wouldn't get thicker still.

Then, shoved round a corner by a bulge of yellow rock, the water whooshed into a tunnel. There were sandy stones either side, but it looked pitch black inside and the boom and rattle of the water and stone was so loud she thought it must destroy her. But she hardly hesitated. Either she followed the water or she died anyway, so she clenched her hands and ducked into the mouth.

*continues*

___ *continued* ___

She felt her way along the tunnel sides, slipping again and again on the rocks and pebbles. But at least it wasn't entirely dark once she was inside, and the noise was unexpectedly invigorating. Ahead she could see a small whitish light which grew as she moved forward. It was the channel's end and before too long she spilled out with the water, falling onto wet earth darkened by giant trees. It was like a second birth.

But the bush would not cradle her. Mungda itched with insect bites and her legs and arms were repeatedly cut as she pushed through the dense plants. She was tiring and crying in frustration.

Then the noise changed. There was the smooth rumble as the river widened alongside her, but there was a deeper sound too — like the thunder when the Big Rain came.

She followed it and soon the bush cleared and she could stand full and watch the water cascade down the cliff below her. It slammed ceaselessly into a great olive-green pool, before running to earth again in the distance, but less madly.

There could be food in the pool. She could live if she could get it.

◆

## MORE RESEARCH NEEDED

Mungda needs to:

a. Detect something edible.
b. Secure something edible.
c. Devour something edible safely.

And she needs more than instinct in order to do any of these things.

If she is to survive she needs a theory capable of identifying something edible in the immediate vicinity. She also needs a theory to enable her to trap something edible, if that something is not passively there for her. And to eat safely she either needs existing knowledge or a way of discovering knowledge.

Mungda must add to her stock of theory by doing research and acting on it – and she must do so soon, before it is too late.

◆

*V*

Mungda climbed a waterside tree to gaze into the pool. She saw what she hoped she would. Fish − plentiful fish − hanging and occasionally swimming just below the surface, out in the centre of the pool. They might be edible, but she hadn't seen this sort of fish before. The fish she knew were small and black and lived in the crashing salt. These were huge and greeny brown with massive bog eyes.

She tried to wade in without disturbing them. As far as she could tell they stayed put beneath the glistening surface, but the water was too deep to reach them. She was not a fish, so she couldn't get to them. She needed to find a way.

She looked around. She noticed birds flying overhead, occasionally settling on the water. She saw insects buzzing, hovering above the surface. She couldn't do those things either. She looked again. There were sticks and leaves and some branches floating in the pool. Could she do the same?

She tried to lay on the water like a leaf, but she sank, arms thrashing, choking water. It was shockingly cold and her nose sucked it in. She crawled out muddily. No good. But maybe if she held onto some sticks? She tried and again she sank, losing grip of the sticks in the process. A larger branch then? She walked along the rim of the pool and came across part of a fallen tree. It was very heavy but she pushed it in and held on. It supported her and she found that if she kicked her legs and held on to the fat stub of a branch she could move slowly across the pool.

◆

## PROVISIONAL RESEARCH RESULTS

Here's how Mungda's research project has continued:

1. It looks like there's food in the water.
   **A hypothesis.**

2. It is not accessible from the bank.
   **An observed fact.**

3. It is possible for some objects to float.
   **A theory based on observation.**

4. It may be possible for me to float. More specifically, if I mimic the leaf I will float in the water.
   **Another hypothesis.**

5. I sank.

   **An experimental result which adds to Mungda's knowledge even though she was wrong.**

6. Larger objects that float may support me.

   **A hypothesis based on intelligent observation.**

7. The sticks fail, but the log carries me in the water.

   **The hypothesis tested, giving an experimental result and some support for Mungda's theory.**

8. Perhaps not all large logs will do this for me but at least this one does.

---

◆

---

## VI

Trying not to splash, Mungda propelled the log toward the area where the fish were basking in the afternoon sunlight. They didn't move away so she lay with one arm on the log looking down at them shimmering in the green. Now she had to catch one. She could not afford to mess this up.

Though the pool was tranquil enough in the middle, the waterfall's boom drummed her ears and the spray reached across the pool to douse her lightly, as the breeze caught it. She was stiffening with the cold and could feel her legs being pulled in the direction of the escaping water. She would have to get it right first time.

You couldn't catch the black fish by the tail so she supposed you couldn't catch these that way either. So she decided to reach underneath one of them to try to throw it up out of the water, onto the log. With luck it would die there.

Slowly she edged her hand forward, until she was beneath the belly of a big one. Then she shot her arm up. The water frothed. The fish flew. But it landed way beyond the log, and darted into the deep.

The other fish scattered, but fortunately for Mungda they didn't go far and soon came back to the middle. Life had been easy for these chubby fish.

If she had something to catch the fish in it wouldn't be so hard. But she didn't, and she couldn't think how to make a trap either. She was so hungry now, and going strangely numb.

She looked at the fish again, panicking briefly. What if I can't get one? I don't want to die like this. I don't want to fail like this. Then she quieted. There must be a way. But how?

With a huge effort of imagination she wondered whether she might not be able to grab hold of one after all. The fish were bigger and slower than the blackfish, and the one she'd touched felt rough and scaly — not smooth like the blackfish. She should try to grab one. She didn't think she could but then she couldn't think of anything else either. And she knew she was weakening. This might be her last chance.

*continues*

— *continued* —

Again she edged her hand forward. Again the fish ignored her. She held her hand open under the back end of one of the smaller ones, one she could get her hand fully round. Then she grabbed and squeezed. And plucked the thing out. Wildly she smashed it against the tree, squeezing so hard her nails sliced painlessly into the ball of her thumb.

The fish lay twitching, its face smashed against the rough wood. Mungda shoved it into a hollow in the trunk so there was no chance it could flip out. She groped round to the other side of the tree and kicked and barged it back to shore.

There was one thing left to do. As hungry as she was she couldn't eat the fish without knowing if it would poison her. She knew that not all fruit and not all animals are safe to eat. She guessed it would be the same with fish so she needed to perform another experiment.

Usually they did it with the dogs. If a dog ate new food and was alright the next day then a few of the older women would try it, and if they were alright then the rest of them would eat. But there was only Mungda, so she needed her ingenuity once again.

She skinned the fish as best she could with icy hands, removing its bones and gut, as they did with the blackfish. She wrapped the white meat in some big leaves to keep it safe, then spread the skin and bones in the hollow of the trunk. She pushed it into the lake and waited.

Almost immediately there were excited cries from the trees, and such a beat of wings that she could feel their wind on her face. With screech on screech the whole flock of them descended on the trunk. There was momentary clamour – wings and beaks dashing into a white and yellow blur – and then it was all gone. The birds glided up to the trees and the hollow was quite empty.

The fish must swim too low for the birds to catch, but they know what a dead one tastes like, she thought. Her heart beating in warm exhilaration Mungda carefully unwrapped her meal, and with a wave to the birds began to eat.

## SECTION TWO

# MUNGDA'S INSPIRATION FOR NURSING RESEARCH

Research is:

**Any method, applied to any phenomenon, that can produce a greater understanding of that phenomenon.**

According to this broad interpretation you can research theological matters, research your thoughts, become expert in astrology, learn philosophical theory, discover a city's cafés, understand your spouse more deeply, study a patient's family background – or find a fish to save your life. Reading a novel, watching a play, listening to your mother, baring your soul – all this can be research if you do it seeking to increase your understanding of the world.

Research in the broadest sense is both science and art, so it is not always necessary to produce testable hypotheses, and there is no requirement to study only the physical world. If a person is exploring some phenomenon in a way she believes might lead to greater understanding then research is going on. Anyone who deliberately attempts to do this is a researcher (which means that every inquisitive nurse is a researcher).

## VALUES INSPIRE RESEARCH GOALS, RESEARCH GOALS SHOULD INSPIRE RESEARCH QUESTIONS

Nurses ought to undertake research inspired by nursing values, for the following reasons.

### 1. Research Is a Basic Feature of Sentient Life
Mungda's story demonstrates that in order to carry out research any researcher needs:

  i. **A question**
  ii. **A method likely to produce an answer to her question.**

This is true of all research, from advanced calculation in higher mathematics to reading a train timetable.

### 2. If Her Research Is to be Meaningful, a Researcher Must Have At Least One Reason to Undertake It
**Research cannot be done arbitrarily. A 'researcher' setting out to 'research' randomly, for no reason, would:**

  a. **Be unable to differentiate between important and useless material.** You can tell the difference between relevant and irrelevant data only if there is some point in your collecting it. If you look at a train timetable for no other reason than it happens to be in front of you, its information will be worthless to you.
  b. **Be unable to decide intelligently when to stop collecting data.** Since the data collection would be arbitrary the researcher would have no means other than whim to decide when to cease her 'inquiries'.

### 3. A Researcher's Reason for Undertaking a Particular Inquiry Must Stem From a Judgement about What Is Important
However scientific the research method, the ultimate reason for pursuing a particular question will be one or more human preference (the evidence does not speak for itself – human beings decide whether what they see is worth investigating[7]).

This is a double-edged sword. A judgement of what is useful or otherwise valuable is required in order to identify a subject to research – yet the same set of beliefs can obscure other understandings of what is useful or otherwise valuable. Notice, for example, how Mungda's judgement about what was useful both helped and restricted her observations and thinking.

Mungda's need to research a source of food enabled her to focus on her primary problem. But her determination to find an answer to this single problem had the effect of shutting off her mind to almost everything else around her. If Mungda had been interested in mapping the forest region rather than searching for food in it she would have seen it differently. Rather than concentrating on the river alone she would have had to make comprehensive observations of shape and contour. The river would have been one feature amongst many, whereas it was all that mattered to the hungry Mungda.

If Mungda had possessed modern knowledge of botany countless food sources would have been available to her. If she had been expert in ornithology she would have been able to ask questions about the eggs of many sorts of bird. If she had known the hibernating habits of sub-tropical rainforest creatures – and how to identify their food stores – she would have been able to frame her inquiry differently again. And if she had needed medicine rather than food she would have asked another set of questions. But her knowledge of what could be eaten was limited, so she saw salvation only in the river, and her questions and methods related to that stretch of water alone.

### 4. Goals Should Be First, Questions Second
Mungda's goal determined the questions she asked. But this is not the only relationship between research goal and research question. It is also possible for a researcher's questions to determine her goals.

In principle, the former is a desirable state of affairs while the latter is not.

    a. **A researcher's questions will be shaped by her goals**. If the researcher says: nursing's mission is to achieve **dignity, ethics and caring relationships** and she can specify what **dignity, ethics and caring relationships** mean in the context of her chosen research area, then **nursing will be in charge of the research process**. The researcher's questions, definition of problem or subject matter, observations, theories, hypotheses and experiments will be guided by nursing's goals (so long as both questions and goals are clearly understood and stated).

    b. **A researcher's goals may be shaped by her questions**. How might this happen?
       Even in her extreme need it might have been possible for Mungda to have asked questions that shaped her search for food differently, or even diverted her from its pursuit altogether.
       Mungda believed the sun is a god and should be worshipped, and that her ancestors were watching over her. Instead of asking: 'Where can I find food?' Mungda might have asked: 'Which sacrifice should I offer up to the sun?' She might have acted on the theory that if she could appease the sun god then she would be saved. Her research programme might then either have been to offer sacrifices and prayers on a trial and error basis, or to try to recall which of the tribe's many rituals would be most effective in the circumstances. If her trawl through her memory led her to conclude that she must sacrifice a large green and red bird (for instance) then she would have had to pursue a supplementary research project: where can I find, catch and sacrifice such a bird in this place?
       Food would still have been the primary goal as Mungda asked: 'Which sacrifice should I offer up to the sun?', but her research questions would

have been directed toward other goals first, and might in the end have caused her to neglect her first goal.

Mungda's research questions may even have caused her not to ask: 'Where can I find food?' For example, she may have decided that she was for some reason being punished by the sun god and would inevitably die soon. Believing this, the only question to occur to her might have been: 'What have I done wrong?' (in fact she had done nothing wrong – she had been deserted because she had not borne any children). She could have devoted her remaining hours to trying to understand what she had done, and in offering prayers to her god to ask her to be merciful.

It could be argued that whatever Mungda's goal, it would still have been in charge of her research. But the point is that her religious questions might have been so powerful as to blind her to her more obvious human goal – to eat as quickly as possible. The questions 'How can I appease the god?' and 'What have I done wrong?' would have overwhelmed her drive to survive.

## THE VACUUM EFFECT

Researchers are not always in control of their research. If a researcher does not have a strong sense of her own purpose then there can be a vacuum effect. Other people's ideas and goals – and sometimes even random ideas – can rush in to possess the research.

Furthermore, the **vacuum effect** tends to have the effect of reinforcing existing priorities, since it is always easier to do what is conventional. It does so:

### 1. By Diverting Attention from Innovative Research Possibilities
If some problems are being researched and others are not then those under scrutiny are more likely to be considered important.

### 2. By Giving the Impression that What is Not Being Researched is Acceptable – that what is not under study is less of a problem simply because it is not presently being investigated.
For example, to carry out only technical research (perhaps into cost-containment, or into how to work a new machine most effectively) in a system that has undergone extensive ideological change is tacitly to approve of the ideological changes by leaving them unexamined. This is the situation in New Zealand, where there has been extensive change in the funding and administration of the health system.[66] Various research projects have been funded by government over the reform period (since 1991) but – unsurprisingly – not one has been commissioned into the merits of the ideological inspiration for the changes.

### 3. By Making it Difficult – if not Impossible – to Carry Out Research into Alternatives to the Existing Ethos
Without a powerful and clearly stated set of purposes (such as those contained in the **Universal Code** – see **Chapter 10**) a sustained and widespread alternative research programme is unlikely to happen.

More specifically, the **vacuum effect** can result in:

a. **Research for research's sake**. Projects done for no other reason than that 'nurses ought to do research' and/or projects which replicate already completed research.

b. **Researching in line with someone else's purpose**. Like other health care researchers, nurse researchers are vulnerable to exploitation through no fault of their own. Nurses keen to research may be able to get funding only for projects sponsored by commercial companies with commercial interests, may be permitted only to carry out certain types of research within hospitals and health authorities, may be under the control of ethics committees with their own purposes, or may be forced to do commissioned studies not in keeping with nursing's true aims.

   If she is in a specialist research department the sorts of project a nurse might get involved in will usually be tightly restricted by precedent. The department might conduct research only into certain aspects of diabetes, or obstetrics, or psychiatric conditions, for instance. Even if the department's research projects are not tightly specified it is likely that the staff will strongly favour some projects over others. Some innovation may be possible, but only within the general departmental ethos.

c. **Research to increase the status of the nursing profession**. The desire for better status can put pressure on nurses to undertake research for reasons other than to acquire useful knowledge:

> Nurses increasingly recognize the need to extend the base of nursing knowledge as part of professional responsibility and endorse scientific investigations as a way to achieve this objective. Moreover, nurses are committed to the evolution of a fairly distinct body of knowledge that separates nursing from other professions. Nursing is only one of several professions involved in the delivery of health care. Information from nursing investigations helps to define better the unique role that nursing plays.[61]

Similar sentiments are widely expressed in the nursing literature. Yet the purposes to extend knowledge and simultaneously to define nursing's 'unique role' are uneasy bedfellows.

The problem is that if nursing research is guided primarily by nursing's wish to become a profession then this will affect research goals – as it would have were Mungda to have tried to appease the sun god.

## THE SUB-HIERARCHY OF NURSING RESEARCH

Nurse researchers should be aware of an important hierarchy:

1. **the goal**
2. **the questions**
3. **the method**

Get this hierarchy wrong and there will be problems. If the hierarchy looks like this:

1. **the method**
2. **the questions**
3. **the goal**

the research will be done for the wrong reason – for instance, because a method is possible and a researcher wants to use it. In this case the questions and the goal become subservient to the method.

If the hierarchy looks like this:

1. **the questions**
2. **the goal**
3. **the method**

then the **vacuum effect** may apply (they may be somebody else's questions).

This is the only way the hierarchy makes sense:

1. **the goal**
2. **the questions**
3. **the method**

This arrangement rightly makes the researcher's own reasons for doing research the first priority. In case it is not obvious why this is so important consider the following situation:

> Three nurses embark on three research projects. The **first nurse** has no interest in her topic (which is on the difference between nurse-monitored and doctor-monitored blood pressure readings) but decides to do it because her employer looks favourably on staff who research. The **second nurse** is interested in finding ways to encourage people to opt out of treatment, in order to reduce waiting lists. She sets up a pilot project to evaluate the performance of a patient questionnaire designed to find out to what extent elderly people are willing to sacrifice their interests for those of younger patients. The **third nurse** wants to know how best to turn nurse theorists' ideas on the importance of dignity into reality on the wards.
>    There is no difference in the quality of the research method each nurse chooses to use. However, there are obvious differences in their motivations – the **first** is doing it for selfish ends, and the **second** for inegalitarian ends. Only the **third** is motivated by a wish to find a way to improve conditions for everyone.

If attention is focused only (or even mostly) on **'are these good research questions?'** or **'is this a good method?'** (Is this a good questionnaire? Is this likely to produce a significant result? Is this reliable and valid?) then something has gone morally askew. The first research question should always be: **what is the point of this research and is it morally justifiable?**

## SUMMARY

Nursing research should be governed by nursing's basic goals (explained in **Chapters Nine** and **Ten**) – the spirit of nursing should guide all nurse researchers. But there are **two obstacles**: nursing's purpose is rarely stated sufficiently explicitly to guide research initiatives, and other purposes keep getting in the way of research based wholly on nursing values.

The final chapters of this book address the first problem. **Section Three** of this chapter suggests one way in which nurses might deal with the second.

*SECTION THREE*

# THE HONEST RESEARCHER TEST

It is widely acknowledged that a researcher should be honest about the strength and weaknesses of his method, should not distort his results and should have read and understood all his sources. It is less often remarked that a researcher should be honest about his motivations, his prejudices, his social and political influences, and his personal feelings about the results he gets.

The **Honest Researcher Test** can help in all these respects (and it is relevant to all researchers, not just nurses). The **Test** is comprised of a series of questions – each of which requires a wholly honest answer. If the researcher is able to complete the **Test** candidly it may be of personal help during a research project.

The **Test** is also valuable as a public declaration, and potential nurse researchers are urged to complete and if possible publish it (amongst their colleagues at least) before they undertake any research. Because so many nurses wish to express their values and are prepared to work according to them, nursing is well placed both to adopt and promote the **Honest Researcher Test**.

As you read the **Test** you may consider it unlikely that it will ever be widely used. If so it may be worth considering why it is so unlikely (what does this say about most current health care research?).

---

### THE HONEST RESEARCHER TEST

Note: This version of the **Honest Researcher Test** is written for nurse researchers.

This test should be completed shortly before a nurse prepares a research application, accepts a research grant and begins a research project. The nurse should be open about the results of the **Test** and should be prepared to change her mind as she considers the results.

*continues*

---

— *continued* —

*SECTION ONE*

## MOTIVATION

### QUESTIONS

### A. WHY DO I WANT TO DO THIS RESEARCH?

**I want to do this research because:**     **TICK APPROPRIATE BOXES. YOU MAY CHOOSE MORE THAN ONE**

1. I want to see if I can find patterns and explanations because (like a child) I am curious to know more for curiosity's sake alone ☐

2. I want to see if I can find patterns and explanations because I think I will be able to put these results to good use ☐

3. I have to see if I can find patterns and explanations because this is what I am employed to do ☐

4. I have to see if I can find patterns and explanations because my employer/funder hopes to be able to put these results to further use ☐

5. I want to do this research for ends other than the research project itself:

    i. I want to get a paper published ☐

    ii. I want to secure research funding ☐

    iii. I want to further the reputation of my profession ☐

    iv. It will help the political cause I support ☐

    v. Some other reason (say what it is ......) ☐

6. Cultural and social expectations (my own and other people's) are pressuring me to go down this research path. In particular, these expectations are:

a.
b.
c. .......

**CAREFULLY SURVEY THIS INFORMATION. IS YOUR JUSTIFICATION FOR DOING THIS RESEARCH ADEQUATE? EVEN IF YOU THINK IT IS, CONTINUE WITH THE TEST**

### B. WHAT ALTERNATIVE RESEARCH COULD I DO?

**List as many alternatives as you can think of – however unlikely they seem.**

**Instead of my proposed project I could do the following:**

a.
b.
c.
d. etc. ......

*continues*

— *continued* —

**Then choose from the possibilities below (you can choose more than one).**

**I have decided not to do the above because:**

   i. I am not technically competent to do a, b, c etc. ☐

  ii. a, b, c etc. are less interesting ☐

 iii. a, b, c etc. are less intellectually challenging ☐

 iv. a, b, c etc. are less likely to be productive ☐

  v. a, b, c etc. are more commonplace ☐

 vi. a, b, c etc. are personally unacceptable ☐

 vii. a, b, c etc. are unacceptable to my colleagues ☐

viii. a, b, c etc. are unacceptable to my employer ☐

 ix. a, b, c etc. are unacceptable to my funder ☐

  x. a, b, c etc. are politically unacceptable ☐

 xi. a, b, c etc. are too risky to me – if I do these then I may damage myself ☐

 xii. I cannot get funding for a, b, c ☐

xiii. Some other reason (say what it is ....)

**ARE THESE GOOD REASONS? IF YOU DO NOT HAVE A GOOD REASON NOT TO DO THE ALTERNATIVES, WHY ARE YOU CHOOSING TO DO YOUR PROPOSED RESEARCH INSTEAD?**

**C. WILL MY RESEARCH FIND ANSWERS THAT ARE ALREADY WELL KNOWN?**

Yes/No

(Note: A day in any university library, perusing any subject, will reveal gross replication of idea and study. Occasionally truly original studies are undertaken, but they are rare and then frequently copied.)

**D. I HAVE CHOSEN THIS RESEARCH METHOD BECAUSE:**

   i. It is most likely to produce a significant result ☐

  ii. I have been told to use it ☐

 iii. It is available ☐

 iv. It is fashionable ☐

  v. I can do it ☐

 vi. I know someone who can help me do it ☐

vii. I have a computer program that can do it ☐

— *continues* —

*— continued —*

**E. I WILL ACCEPT AND TRY TO PUBLISH WHATEVER RESULT I ACHIEVE, EVEN IF:**

i.    It is not what I predicted ☐

ii.   It seems to make further research projects less attractive ☐

iii.  It is not the result I wanted ☐

iv.   It is not the result my employer wanted ☐

v.    It is not the result my funder wanted ☐

vi.   It places me in danger of ridicule or some other personal harm ☐

**HAVING ANSWERED A TO E OF SECTION ONE YOU SHOULD BE IN A POSITION TO COMPLETE THE FOLLOWING STATEMENT CANDIDLY:**

**I AM CHOOSING TO DO THIS RESEARCH BECAUSE**

...........................................................................................................

...........................................................................................................

...........................................................................................................

...........................................................................................................

...........................................................................................................

...........................................................................................................

...........................................................................................................

*SECTION TWO*

## GUIDING PHILOSOPHY

**A. HAVE I SAID: 'I AM CHOOSING TO DO THIS RESEARCH BECAUSE I BELIEVE ITS GOALS ARE THE MOST IMPORTANT I COULD POSSIBLY AIM FOR'?**

YES/NO

**B. IF NO, WHY NOT?**

...........................................................................................................

...........................................................................................................

...........................................................................................................

**C. IF YES:**

i.    What are these goals?

...........................................................................................................

...........................................................................................................

*continues —*

--- *continued* ---

..........................................................................................
..........................................................................................
..........................................................................................

ii. Are the ends of my research project consistent with the nursing values I have committed to?

YES/NO/DON'T KNOW

**D. HOW LIKELY IS IT THAT MY RESEARCH WILL PRODUCE RESULTS THAT WILL CONVINCE OTHERS TO ACT IN LINE WITH NURSING VALUES?**

i.   Unlikely ☐
ii.  Probable ☐
iii. Certain ☐
iv.  Unpredictable ☐

**E. ARE THERE BETTER WAYS OPEN TO ME TO BRING ABOUT CHANGE IN LINE WITH THE GOALS OF NURSING I HAVE COMMITTED TO?**

..........................................................................................
..........................................................................................
..........................................................................................

Once the nurse has answered the **Test** honestly she should be in a stronger position to decide honestly whether to write her proposal, accept a research grant or begin a research project than she was before.

The best nursing research requires two elements: the researcher should be ruthlessly honest about her motivations and should base her research on a clear philosophy of nursing. Done properly the **Honest Researcher Test** ensures the first requirement, and provides some progress toward the latter.

*SECTION FOUR*

# NURSING RESEARCH SHOULD BE BASED ON NURSING VALUES

## AN EXAMPLE: CARING RESEARCH

**We have established that**:

1. We are all researchers.
2. Our judgements about what is important can both enable and restrict our research.

3. There are many reasons for doing research – some commendable and some questionable.
4. Since nursing is trying to develop an ethical form of practice (often in circumstances that are less than morally ideal) it makes sense to base nursing research on nursing values – and to do first those projects likely to further those values in practice.

For example, assuming that advocacy in the **normal sense** is a nursing value (it is a **secondary purpose** on the nursing hierarchy explained in **Chapters Nine** and **Ten**), research could be done to understand more about its effects on patients and nurses, or to learn more about how to advocate effectively (examples of projects undertaken can be found elsewhere[67,68]).

Caring is also a suitable research topic (it is a **primary purpose** on the nursing hierarchy explained in **Chapter Nine**). In 1986 the journal *Topics in Clinical Nursing* ran a theme issue on caring, introduced like this:

> While caring may sound soft or unscientific to some, there are nurse scholars who have begun to study caring scientifically, both from descriptive and experimental approaches...
>
> For nurses to move caring into the arena of scientific investigations shows daring and indicates that 'nursing research' is coming more of age. Indeed, caring actions can be intentionally performed and their effects on patients' welfare documented...
>
> Examining the absence of caring may lead to better understanding of its presence. Often caring involves interactive behaviours such as listening and touching. Investigation of these behaviours could lead to scientific documentation that caring is clinically effective as an intervention...
>
> The phenomenon of caring is a rich source of research for nurses.[69]

## AREAS OF INTEREST

There are already several examples of this type of nursing research.[70,71] To increase the chances of similar projects in future **caring research** might be divided into separate areas of interest. For example:

1. **Research into how to care better** (i.e. direct work with patients and those close to them to discover how to deliver the different **types of care** – see **Chapter Three** – optimally).
2. **Research into how to design and assess health policy in line with a philosophy of care** (i.e. work to devise and assess health policies, either to see whether existing policies are caring or to discern the effectiveness of policies explicitly designed to care).
3. **Other research inspired by notions of care** (i.e. work to introduce **the care factor** into planning research of other kinds – for example, needs assessment or curriculum design).

The **first** requirement of **caring research** is a well-defined understanding of what care and caring is (see **Chapter Three**). The **second** is a comprehensive set of questions about caring – what do we need to know to advance our understanding of care? The **third** is to devise ways to answer these questions, and the **fourth** is to assess their strength.

The **areas of interest** above might be elaborated as follows (note that these are meant as illustrative possibilities only – they are obviously not properly formulated research proposals, and numerous additional ideas are possible).

## Research into How to Care Better

*Possible Studies*

There is probably no end to the number of ways a researcher might investigate **how to care better**. One might, for example:

i. **Offer patients different understandings of care (the different versions outlined in Chapter Three, for example) to discover (through interview) what care means for them, and what their preferences for practical care are.**

ii. **Offer specific groups of patients different understandings of care in order to discover whether different groups have different preferences.**

    For example, geriatric patients, patients who have experienced intensive care, cancer patients and mentally ill patients might be researched to see whether they understand 'care' differently, and also to discover what their practical need for care is (do they, for instance, require nurses first to 'take care' to do a good technical job or do they rank 'emotional involvement' most highly instead?).

iii. **Investigate the physical and emotional effect of different forms of caring, in matched and controlled trials.**

    For example, a nurse researcher might take a group of patients with a similar level of multiple sclerosis who require respite care, and design programmes of care based on the **four types of care** identified in **Chapter Three**.

    The nature of these **types**, and the activities they permit and exclude, could be carefully defined, and experiments could proceed. One group could receive one type of care for a month, another group a different form and so on, after which the groups could be assessed for any number of dependent variables (Are there significant physical differences? Are there differences in affect? How did the patients enjoy their time? Would they want to be cared for like this in future? Have their relationships with their full-time carers now changed?).

    Similar experiments might be conducted with different sets of patients – chronically sick children, the mentally ill, regular general practice patients – in order to construct a more general picture of the effects of different ways of caring.

iv. **Experiments might be conducted in which doctors care in one way and nurses care in another (in a controlled trial).**

    Then the roles could be reversed in order to discover the extent to which patient expectations and perceptions of role make a difference to the effect of care.

v. **Caring can involve tangible actions such as listening, touching, responding thoughtfully to questions, and conversing relevantly. These behaviours might be investigated – in various ways and settings – in order to test the hypothesis that doing them can be clinically effective.**

    For example, in specialist Alzheimer's units with much higher numbers of staff than the norm, it is possible to spend constructive time with patients and so do away with most of the drugs considered necessary in less well-resourced situations.[72] Most nurses and doctors know that hugs are better than drugs in such situations, but are not presently in a position to make this the rule by carrying out influential research.

vi. **Some nurses are better at caring than others. Tests to identify the 'most caring' nurses could be devised.**

This type of nurse could be found and further investigations could begin. Are female nurses more caring than male nurses? Is caring intuitive? Is it a personality trait? Is it learnt? Does caring require a deliberate effort? What is the effect of insisting that professional nurses carry out caring behaviours whether they mean them or not? What enables caring and what prohibits it?

No doubt these studies pose many challenges of research design – possibly even insuperable difficulties – but no matter, there are many alternatives (What are the effects on carers of caring in different ways? What are the financial implications? Are there other economic considerations? Can caring attitudes be educated? What are the legal implications of favouring emotional commitment above technical wizardry?). The crucial point is that it is possible to design studies explicitly in line with a central nurse value.

## Research into How to Design and Assess Health Policy in Line with a Philosophy of Care

'Health reforms' are frequently introduced on the assumption they will improve services, despite the absence of an assessment of the benefits and disadvantages of the existing system.[66] Once implemented they are rarely analysed to see whether the predicted improvements have occurred.[73]

One of the reasons for this lack of rigour is – as always – that the necessary denominators ('health gain', 'efficiency', 'value for money' and so on) are not sufficiently well defined to permit testable hypotheses (too often they are not even defined at all[74]).

By contrast, nursing might lead the way in **health reform research** and so promote kinder health systems. Nursing could do this by defining indicators of care, assessing current health systems to see the extent to which these indicators are present, suggesting reforms to health systems based on these indicators, and then comparing the systems before and after the reforms.

The central question would be: **is the reformed system more caring than the old one?**

*Possible Studies*

i. **The extent to which 'caring practice' takes place in current health systems could be reviewed.**

ii. **The information could be compared to analogous information (where available) from previous health systems.**

(Is there more or less care now? Is it possible to detect the impact of change in caring on patients and staff?).

iii. When reform is next suggested nurses would be able to run pilot studies to discover whether proposed changes would improve caring practice or not.

iv. If it becomes widely agreed that 'being taken seriously', 'being listened to', 'being involved in decision-making' form part of caring practice then these may constitute good reasons for nurses to want to suggest reform programmes of their own.

Nurses might carry out pilot studies of parts of health systems in which there is a deliberate and clearly defined attempt to increase democratic participation (perhaps involving all staff equally in decision-making). They might then make use of the results (whatever they are) to argue for policy changes.

## Other Research Inspired by Notions of Care

*Possible Studies*

i. Adding a 'caring dimension' to existing projects currently lacking one.

An example in this category might be a needs assessment exercise in which patients are asked fixed questions, but are not yet asked about whether they want to be 'taken seriously', 'given comprehensive information', 'provided with a nurse who will endeavour to become emotionally attached to them', and so on.

Another example might be whether to offer patients the opportunity not only to participate in clinical trials in which they will be randomly assigned to a new drug, a placebo or a control group, but where they can – if they want to take the risk – try out the new drug anyway (on the ground that this respects them fully and is therefore typically caring).[75] If patients were to be offered this chance a further avenue for research – the study of these people's reactions to being so trusted – would open up.

ii. Adding a 'caring dimension' to new projects to examine phenomena and treatments.

An example in this category might assess the treatment of patients in 'acute in-patient mental health units'. Treatment in these units is often based on power and coercion – a **caring research** project might examine the effect of engaging patients in partnership and co-operation (for example, by giving non-dangerous patients the combination to the locks protecting secure wards).

*Limitations of Situation*

It must be said, once again, that practical matters severely limit innovative projects such as these. Most clinical nurses do not have sufficient time for research. Indeed, they rarely have enough time to care as much as they would like in the present climate, in which governments and health managers are obsessed with cost-reduction. Furthermore, at the moment research is mostly done by those (short-term students or academics) who do not necessarily value caring as highly as practising nurses, and who do not have to implement policies based on their research.

But though this is the way things are, it is no reason not to try to bring change about.

## CONCLUSION

I am suggesting that nursing wear its heart on its sleeve and that the leaders of the profession loudly and consistently proclaim that a central aspect of what nurses do is

**caring research** (and other research based on nursing values as outlined in **Chapter Nine**). Nursing research should become synonymous with research based on the purposive system explained in **Chapters Nine** and **Ten**.

Before researching anything, a nurse must ask: **what does my commitment to nursing inspire me to research?** Only if she can answer this fundamental question should she ask: **by what method can I find out what I want to know?**

# CHAPTER SEVEN

# Ethics

## SUMMARY

This chapter:

1. Offers a brief account of **the ethics of care** (an approach favoured by many nurse theorists).
2. Argues that the **defence of tenderness** is **caring ethics'** most important contribution.
3. Shows what can happen when clinical work is done in the absence of tenderness.
4. Describes a **solely analytic response** to a nursing problem.
5. Shows that the **analytic response** fails primarily because it denies the importance of values.
6. Describes a **solely caring response** to a nursing problem.
7. Shows that **caring ethics** alone is not enough to solve the problem.
8. Expounds an approach which unites analysis and caring.

◆

---

### *CASE FIVE*

### Stephanie's Problem

Stephanie is a young nurse, only recently qualified. She enters a four-bedded surgical ward to administer a round of medication. A patient to her left is groaning loudly, in obvious pain. In the opposite bed an elderly man lies deeply asleep. Another — older still — stares blankly at the scudding sky outside, moist eyes frozen in a snowy face.

Even before Stephanie is through the door the fourth patient starts to shout, gesturing in agitation toward the groaning man. 'Get him to shut up can't you nurse? He's driving me mad. Get him out of here or get him sedated. I can't take any more.'

## INTRODUCTION

Nurses regularly encounter situations like this. They are not necessarily 'life and death' crises, but always require careful handling if they are to be resolved well. Nurse theorists urge nurses to adopt **the ethics of care** in order to deal with them. They say this is the deepest possible moral response, and unique to nursing.

**Section One** of this chapter explains nurse theorists' opposition to orthodox moral reasoning, and outlines their alternative. It also describes a solely analytic response and a solely caring response to Stephanie's problem, and shows that each is inadequate on its own.

**Section Two** demonstrates how nursing might combine tenderness with intelligent analysis – and so lead the way in ethical analysis in health care.

*SECTION ONE*

## THE ETHICS OF CARE

## WHY NURSE THEORISTS ADVOCATE NURSING ETHICS

Nurse theorists regularly remark that nurses are about to come up with an original way of dealing with ethical matters:

> '. . . it is important to . . . claim the right to use the term nursing ethics. Nursing is a separate discipline from the other professions involved in health care, and therefore we bring our own issues, concerns, problems and dilemmas into a health care arena in which we as nurses need to look for and work out a resolution.[56]

> . . . ethics can no longer be viewed only from the . . . philosophical traditions of the western world . . . a model for nursing ethics that is context-sensitive, rather than universal in nature, needs to be developed.[76]

Nursing's quest for a new type of ethics grew out of opposition to doctors' moral inflexibility, and dissatisfaction with bioethicists' preoccupation with universal principles:

> . . . (nurse theorists disliked) the way in which the impersonal, logical, sterile ways of the modern hospital seemed to be mirrored in the impartial, intellectual logic of modern biomedical ethics. Nursing ethicists realised that this impartiality was not necessarily a feature of good nursing or medical care, where the ultimate value of encounters often seems to rest in the individual human contact between patients and their carers rather than in the intellectualism of diagnosis and treatment . . . nurses could not identify with the medical profession and indeed often felt that they were acting in opposition to the technological aspects of medical care . . .
>   In a famous paper that looked at women who were making decisions about abortions, Gilligan found that many women did not regard morality in terms of justice and competing rights but instead saw it in terms of the need to nurture and maintain human relationships involving emotional responses to the concrete details of particular situations . . . Gilligan therefore claimed that women had a 'care focus' in moral reasoning that had been ignored or underplayed . . . (Gilligan, 1982[77])

Gilligan's ideas about an ethics of care strongly influenced the views of many nurse-ethicists who saw them as providing a viable alternative to the dominance of principle-based ethics (Davis, 1985[78]).[25]

## WHAT TO DO TO CARE ETHICALLY

According to the care-oriented approach, in order to care ethically a nurse **should**:

1. Respond directly – as a part of the situations she encounters. The ethical nurse should immerse herself in her patients' worlds, achieving empathy spontaneously, by reacting to their moods and behaviour without pretence.
2. Ideally, the ethical nurse should not only establish sincere relationships with her patients, she should become so deeply attached to them that their interests become hers:

> ...[n]ursing is basically being-for-the-other...[79]

At its most intense the idea is that the ethical nurse ought to develop, with every patient:

> ...a kind of indwelling relationship, an engrossment and motivational displacement derived from feminine emotional qualities.[38]

Less extremely, the ethical nurse will exhibit:

> ...four critical attributes... – 'serious attention', 'concern', 'providing for' and 'getting to know the patient'.[80]

by:

> ... listening to others, understanding them, and responding with appreciation of their intentions[81]

## WHAT NOT TO DO

If she is to care ethically a nurse **should not**:

1. Apply general principles (like 'be just', 'respect autonomy' and 'be beneficent') to deal with ethical problems. Unique circumstances merit unique human responses. Applying rules to unpredictable, emotional situations inhibits intuition and corrupts natural relationships.

Nor should she:

2. Analyse situations dispassionately. According to some commentators the ethical nurse should not even work out a strategy of her own. Rather she must:

> ...set aside [her] temptation to analyse and to plan. I do not project; I receive the other into myself, and I see and feel with the other. I become a duality...[38]

It is not always easy to understand why nurse theorists take such an uninhibited stance. Indeed, some analysts have dismissed **the ethics of care** as too vague in theory (what exactly does it mean to 'receive another into myself'?) and too hard in practice (how can I possibly act according to it?).[82,83] Yet nursing's attachment to the **ethics of care** (despite its intellectual deficiencies) is helping to preserve a precious tenderness.

Tenderness is not something one should analyse, though we should try to experience and offer it as often as we can. Tenderness is most obvious in its absence. It is painfully apparent when it is missing, because without it everything becomes disposable – and the ethics of care rightly resists this desolate view of human interaction.

## WHEN TENDERNESS IS ABSENT

There is a perception amongst doctors, bioethicists, and the general public that the great majority of conventional health care is carried out to the highest ethical standards.[84] There may be occasional blips,[9] and there will always be controversies,[85] but health care is generally one of the most – if not the most – honourable of endeavours.

Unfortunately, most nurses know better. Unless they are very lucky they see (and are sometimes part of) daily examples of crass practice performed by professional people accepting – and so perpetuating – unkind traditions without question.

### SOME EXAMPLES

Part of the problem is that too many health professionals overprotect themselves from others' experience, so nullifying tenderness. Here are five cases of **tender-less health care**, taken from a boxful of evidence reported by fifth year medical students in response to my request for reports of 'ethically interesting situations' encountered in clinical departments. Every year, between 20 and 30% of the clinical students divulge similar experiences.

---

**Student 1: Secrets in Oncology**

In the oncology clinic my role was observational. I met Mrs K, 32 years old, who had metastatic breast disease and was receiving palliative care. During the interview it became apparent to me that the patient didn't realise that the treatment option is not a cure and that she will die of her disease in the near future. After she left I raised this issue with the consultant, who replied, 'I don't tell them if they don't ask me.'

---

**Student 2: Informed Consent in ENT**

A diagnosis of malignancy had been made by means of a needle biopsy from a metastatic node in the elderly man's neck. The clinical director asked the patient

*continues*

---

— *continued* —

what he knew of his condition. The patient told him he was anxious to know because nothing had been said. The director told him he had 'a serious growth in his neck' and nothing more regarding prognosis or treatment. It struck me that everyone knew exactly what this man had except the patient himself. He had even received intensive investigation – the needle biopsy – without being told what was being looked for.

I find this situation interesting from the point of view that the law says that for any procedure there must be informed consent – which obviously wasn't obtained prior to the needle biopsy.

---

### Student 3: MS = Poor Quality of Life?

My case involves a 38-year-old woman who had multiple sclerosis. She was living independently at home, with some help from her husband. She walked either on crutches or a 'walker'. She came to hospital with peritonitis – nothing to do with her MS.

She consented to an operation to wash out her abdomen and reconnect her bowel. She was very sick (septic) afterwards, unable to converse – the doctors wanted to move her to the intensive care ward. The intensive care consultant refused to take her on the ground of her MS – she said they do not accept people for intensive care who will not have a good quality of life afterwards (referring to the MS).

The patient stayed on our ward and died two days later.

---

### Student 4: He's a No-hoper Anyway

A 28-year-old Maori man presented at A&E with a chest injury following a car crash in which he was driving drunk. He had a small pneumothorax which didn't warrant treatment and was discharged to the police. The next day he was gaoled. In frustration he pushed his hand through a pane of glass, requiring readmission. A routine chest X-ray showed a complete deflation of his left lung which required urgent re-inflation. The registrar inserted a chest drain, but thought it would make a good teaching case and got his colleagues (a registrar and a house officer) to insert, remove, re-insert, remove, re-insert, remove and re-insert the chest drain.

This was a huge ethical issue for me. The registrar justified his actions by saying 'well ... he was a no-hoper anyway'. But I knew it was wrong. However, it was only through deliberation that I understood why.

---

### Student 5: Public Bad News

I was in an ENT clinic with eight of my fellow medical students one Friday morning. We were expected to go around to various rooms in the outpatient

*continues*

*continued*

clinic, examine each patient and talk to them (I should mention that there was a consultant in the corridor yelling at anyone who wasn't in a consulting room with a patient).

A backup occurred. Either students had to be in a room in numbers in excess of four or out in the hallway being told off by the consultant. Many students responded to this by walking into any room where they saw other students, presumably assuming some sort of global consent from the patients.

Eventually a young man, his mother and grandmother were in a room being told about his cancer and his treatment options with no less than fifteen other people crowded in. At one stage the grandmother offered a student her chair. It was accepted, even though this meant that the grandmother had to leave the room.

It is surely obvious that in each of these cases if the doctor had been the patient he would not have wanted to be treated in this manner. He would want information, he would want his doctor to be aware that 'quality of life' is a subjective judgement, he would want to be protected from pressure and ridicule. He would want kindness, compassion and empathy. He would require tenderness, and if he did not receive it no doubt he would want to know why.

There are many reasons for these ethically barren episodes. One of the easiest to understand is that the idea of getting involved with people – just because they are people – is not discussed and not valued in most medical education and practice.

Nursing clearly knows better. Nursing's understanding of ethics rightly places tenderness at the forefront of clinical work – yet the ethical incompetencies roll on and on, and show no sign of decreasing. And this – it seems to me – ought to act as a massive spur to nursing to:

a. **Understand and explain what is currently wrong.**
b. **Offer a coherent, caring alternative to all health workers.**
c. **Demonstrate how to apply it consistently in practice (i.e. to lead by example).**

Of course this is easier said than done. However nurse theory has got part of the way there already – by taking a concerted stand against **tender-less practice**, and by pointing out that logical analysis is no guarantee of ethical behaviour.

## NURSING'S OPPOSITION TO TENDER-LESS ANALYSIS

Nurse theorists' case is not confined to criticism of isolated examples of **tender-less practice**. They see a more pervasive problem – that **the intellectual approach to ethics is corrupted by the analytic method itself**.

# AN INTELLECTUAL RESPONSE TO STEPHANIE'S PROBLEM

To understand what they mean, imagine someone else – not a nurse but a postgraduate health economist (Andrea) – confronted by the tense situation in the four-bedded ward (see **Case Five** above).

Like Stephanie, the health economist is at first daunted by the intense atmosphere, but keeps panic at bay by asking: **What does my health economics training tell me I should do?** Andrea knows she will first have to define and then work out how to maximise **benefit**, taking account of other benefits she must forgo in the attempt. She must decide whether to maximise happiness, social order, clinical effectiveness, or one of many other possible utilities. And she must also figure out what price she is prepared to pay in order to do it.

Because she is the analyst, and because there is no one else to ask, it falls to Andrea to choose the goal in this case. Surveying the scene from the doorway she defines benefit as 'a calm, therapeutic environment', and considers the situation sufficiently serious to concentrate on.

Andrea chooses to work with a form of utilitarianism[86] that identifies each patient as *prima facie* equally important (each counting as one unit in any calculation). She then tries to assess the level of calmness of each, using notions of 'distress' and 'ability to function according to choice' – each of which she crudely spells out.

She grades the patients numerically in her mind's eye, ranking them on two simple scales:

**Distress Scale 0–10** (where 10 equals 'total peace with the world' and 0 equals 'extreme pain overriding anything else').
**Function Scale 0–10** (where 10 equals 'able to do anything he wants to' and 0 equals 'unable to do anything he wants to').

While obviously limited, this method at least gives Andrea a way to **work out** rather than **feel out** or intuit what to do. She thinks quickly, and hits on a provisional result:

---

**Patient One (The Groaning Man)**

Level of Distress – 2

Level of Function – 0

**Patient Two (The Sleeping Man)**

Level of Distress – 10?, 9? (Is he dreaming?)

Level of Function – 0? 10? (not clear at the moment)

**Patient Three (The Sad Man)**

Level of Distress – 5? 4? (investigation required)

Level of Function – 7? 6? (investigation required)

continues

---

---

— *continued* —

**Patient Four (The Angry Man)**

Level of Distress – 4

Level of Function – 6

---

Andrea needs to check out these ratings – to ask questions to discover if she has read the situation accurately. Ideally she would like to improve each patients' scoring, in the hope of raising the overall scores as close to 80 as possible (she has given the four patients two 10-point scales each), to do so efficiently and at the lowest possible cost.

But now Andrea strikes limits.

---

### A PRACTICAL LIMIT – COMPETENT ANALYSIS TAKES TOO LONG

The trouble with Andrea's method is, first, that it takes too long to do it seriously. In order even to begin her calculations Andrea has already had to define **benefit** and **cost**, and work out an appropriate ranking scale. Now – to do the hard work – she must apply these notions to each of the people directly involved, and possibly to others too as she learns more about the situation.

But to do this much is out of the question in any situation which requires rapid resolution.

---

### A THEORETICAL LIMIT – THE ANALYST MUST MAKE SUBJECTIVE JUDGEMENTS

The second problem is theoretical. However technical her analysis appears – however many numbers she attaches to circumstances and feelings, and however many formulae she uses to work with these numbers – there is no disguising the extent to which human biases must colour her thinking.

The economic method is far more reliant on opinion than it seems at first sight. There is, for example, no objective or value-free way to decide how to define the benefits and costs in this matter – ultimately Andrea must choose in some manner that does not rely on the utilitarian analysis itself. She must either ask the participants to define the costs and benefits themselves, apply hospital rules (if there are any), select randomly, or plump for a utility according to her own preferences.

She is a quiet person, which is why she favours a calm environment. But if she hated discomfort she might have chosen **minimise pain**, if she were gregarious she might have preferred **foster relationships**, if she were a disciplinarian she might have opted for **enforce rules** – there is no end to the targets an analyst might choose.

*continues*

— *continued* —

Furthermore, Andrea has to decide whether to seek a solution which distributes the benefit (a calm, therapeutic environment) equally amongst the four patients, or whether to go for a solution which achieves the highest utility on aggregate. If she chooses the former she will probably find a compromise answer to the problem – an answer that does not achieve the best possible solution for each separate person, but does do so for all of them considered as a unit. If she chooses the latter then she might sort matters out by raising the scores of three of the patients as high as possible, while disregarding or even disadvantaging the other patient. Overall utility will be raised in this way, but at the expense of one of the participants.

Whatever she decides, it is impossible for her to do so other than by making a judgement based on some human value or other. Ethical deliberation can only ever be partly technical – every analysis starts and ends with personal opinion.

## THE ANALYTIC MYTH

Surprisingly there are many (including Andrea's teachers) who do not accept this. They claim their role is merely to provide the basic tools, and that it is for others to say how these tools should be used:

> . . . is (it) appropriate or legitimate to use preferences of the community even if they can be successfully measured . . . (?) Certainly, as economists we would not claim that we can or should determine this but what we would want to investigate is whether the community has a view . . .[87]

> Whose values should count? As a health economist it is not really for me to say. Nor, as a health economist, do I have to say . . .[88]

> Is not the best researcher the 'disinterested' researcher?[89]

Most health economists apparently see themselves as empiricists – as impartial inventors of technical mechanisms, or as field workers seeking merely to discover and respond to the wishes of the public. But – just like any other means of intervening in human affairs – health economics cannot possibly be a value-free enterprise. There is no such thing as a neutral framework or denominator in health economics. Any method of eliciting people's values (short of giving them a blank sheet of paper and asking them to write down anything that occurs to them) will itself be based on values. The economist decides what area to investigate, what health means, what sort of questions to ask, who to ask, when to start and when to stop. The economist's method of calculation does not make these decisions for her – they simply must be human choices.

Take the example of **opportunity cost** employed by Andrea (**opportunity cost** is the benefits one must forgo as one pursues a chosen goal: for example, a cost of my pursuing an opportunity to read a book to my daughter is not being able to work on my own book for a while). Health economists assume that because opportunity cost is an obvious truism, any application of it must also be unarguable. But this is like thinking that because we must all live on a planet where gravity is inescapable, any **use** of gravity must be value-free. And this is blatantly untrue – anyone can see the moral difference between using sledges to slide injured people down mountain-sides and throwing children from tall buildings for sport.

This is not merely a theoretical problem. Every time health economists think they are doing something value-free when they are really making biased choices they reinforce a technically obsessed health system – a system that grossly underestimates the importance of tenderness. For example, a team of health economists recently published an apparently innocuous paper (typical of health economics' contribution to health care)[90] in which they described a project to obtain information from parents about child health services in the Grampian region, North East Scotland. The economists chose to use a willingness to pay (**WTP**) method, as a way to elicit the parents' values. They asked questions such as:

> Would you be willing to pay anything in extra taxation or a voluntary contribution for your child to receive day-case care instead of in-patient care?

> What is the maximum amount that you would be willing to pay over the next 12 months for your child to receive day-case care instead of in-patient care?

They asked them in order to discover the weight of parents' preferences for day-case surgery and overnight stay for tonsillectomy. They also tried to find out parents' preferences for hospital-based clinics and local clinics for bed-wetting, and school health services for all children and only for those with special needs.

The questions, they said:

> ...were framed in such a way as to provide realistic options to the parents[89]

They also explained that:

> The questions reflected choices that the Health Board were [sic] making regarding how it should allocate the limited resources at its disposal between competing causes.[89]

The economists maintain that they were merely carrying out a commission, in a disinterested way – as if they were mathematicians paid to provide a solution to an abstract numerical problem. But it just isn't so.

One need only ask the economists: Would your research programme have been disinterested had the Grampian Board asked you to look into the following issues instead?

> Whether parents accused but not convicted of child abuse should be allowed to see their children at home or in the 'care institution'.

> Whether children should be fitted with electronic tags and tape-recorders and allowed home until the court case, or should always be accompanied by supervisors.

> Whether parents would prefer health service spending on child abuse investigations to be increased, or whether spending should be spread across all children.

If the point is not already plain one might ask a further question: **Would your research be disinterested if you were approached by a military regime interested in gaolers' preferences in regard to three sorts of torture?** Presumably any economist would think very seriously about the hypothetical Grampian programmes – both because these are sensitive matters and because each reflects a debatable way of spending public money. And presumably all honourable economists would refuse to entertain the army's request. But to concede this much is to admit that producing **any** results to meet specific 'information needs' cannot be value-free.

The Scottish economists might respond that there is a marked contrast between their actual project and the additional examples. But though there is an obvious difference in degree of controversy, they would be wrong to think there is a difference in kind. Let's spell it out:

- Deciding to take on the actual Grampian project was to decide not to do all those other things they might have been doing instead (opportunity cost). Some of those things they chose not to do must have been morally worse and some must have been morally better than doing what they did.
- To constrict their research programme as they did (which was admittedly the only way to meet the Grampian board's request) is to do research in an artificial box. It is to say: out of all the services on which parents might be asked to report their willingness to pay, we will inquire only about these. Thus the economists both accept the Grampian board's value-judgement (the board could have commissioned all manner of alternative projects) and make their own judgement that the research is worthwhile (just as they would doubtless judge the torture research not worthwhile).
- To accept this reality (the prevailing state of affairs in the Grampian region) is to accept the status quo, which is a value-judgement regardless of whether you think you can do anything to change it (you don't have to choose to be part of it).
- To accept this reality is to accept the necessity of rationing in the areas on which questions were asked. Each question was an either/or, and gave parents no chance to say, for instance, 'we'd like to see tonsillectomy day surgery expanded *and* more provision for in-patient care'. Thus, by asking these questions the researchers cannot help but add to the climate in which this form of rationing is regarded as inevitable. Their research is, undeniably, a particular social intervention, based on a particular set of values and prejudices.

## NURSING'S PLEA FOR TENDERNESS

Health economists and like-minded policy-makers seem compelled to attach labels to everything – as if they are running a garage sale in which every item must be tagged and priced or no one will buy it. But they define so much so crudely that their classifications corrupt our experience. Their impoverished language creates a parody of the world, concealing what is really important. By so outspokenly opposing this so-called value-neutral approach, nurse theorists do health care an inestimable service. They entreat nurses to care naturally and unashamedly – rightly perceiving that this is the only way health care can retain and expand its sensitivity.

## A NURSING RESPONSE TO STEPHANIE'S PROBLEM

However, though compassionate responses to distress are sometimes all that's needed, most problems require more than this. In Stephanie's case, for example, the caring approach crashes to a halt even more rapidly than the intellectual option.

According to the **ethics of care**, Stephanie must establish relationships with each of the four patients. She must immerse herself in their lives, achieving empathy by reacting to their moods and behaviour without affectation. The ethical nurse should develop '...a kind of indwelling relationship' with every patient – or at the very least must '...listen to others, understand them, and respond with appreciation of their intentions'. Unless she can do these things she cannot possibly care for them in the recommended way – which means that Stephanie immediately faces practical and theoretical barriers.

---

### A PRACTICAL LIMIT – STEPHANIE CAN'T ESTABLISH THE NECESSARY RELATIONSHIPS

The trouble is that one patient is unconscious, one is in great pain, one is angry and one is sad.

In the circumstances it is either impossible or very difficult to establish meaningful relationships. Certainly Stephanie cannot become emotionally attached to the unconscious patient – at least not at this point. And it is unlikely she will quickly be able to establish rapport with any of the others.

---

### A THEORETICAL LIMIT – THERE'S NO PRACTICAL GUIDANCE

However much she feels for the patients – however deeply she understands their plight – her caring presence alone is not enough to solve the problem. None of the exhortations – to 'be-for' patients, to be 'authentically present', to 'self-actualise' and the rest – offer practical guidance to Stephanie.

This is a general problem for the caring approach. Caring ethics offers no help in emotionally awkward situations. For example, **it is not possible simply to care**:

**1. When patients do not want intense involvement**
Several surveys[25] have discovered that not all patients want nurses to throw themselves into their lives. Common experience tells us that we take to some people more than others, and we sometimes find we do not like people – even if they like us.

**2. When emotional involvement does not or cannot achieve the desired result**
Even if she is able to connect emotionally with some of her patients, they will not necessarily see things as the nurse does. Emotional connections are not necessarily

_____ *continues* _____

—— *continued* ——

positive. The nurse and her patients might feel mutual dislike. Or she will discover that she empathises well with some, but resents others (and according to this understanding of ethics she must accept her feelings – **pretend empathy** is unacceptable on the **ethics of care**).

Furthermore, a nurse's response to any situation is bound to be coloured by her upbringing, nationality and educational experience. Nurses' human receptiveness is also likely to be distorted by professional understandings and hospital priorities. 'OK,' Stephanie might say, 'so the **Angry Man** is really fed up, but if he'd seen what I've seen he'd realise it could be a lot worse.' But once a nurse thinks like this she is not empathising – she is projecting, and it is hard to see how she can avoid doing so, at least some of the time.

**3. When discrimination is necessary**
For instance, when the nurse has more than one patient and their needs are either incompatible or cannot be met equally – as in Stephanie's case. It would – from a technical point of view if nothing else – be sensible for Stephanie immediately to establish why the **Groaning Man** is in such pain. Has something happened? Have stitches burst? Is his medication wrong? Is there a clinical crisis?

**4. When other carers, with different ideas about ethics and their professional role, are involved in planning for patients**
Commitment to the ethics of care is not enough to convince those who are not similarly committed.

## HER CARING IS NOT SUFFICIENT TO HELP STEPHANIE FIND AN ETHICAL SOLUTION

She cannot 'be-for' all the patients simply because she cannot make emotional contact with all of them. One cannot become 'a duality' with another person unless one knows the other person. Stephanie might try to act in her patients' best interests, but she will have to guess what these are if her patients cannot or will not tell her – and this is quite different from 'seeing and feeling *with* the other'.

If she can empathise only with those she can 'morally touch'[79] then she will inevitably favour some patients over others – simply because she must be motivated more by the grief of the patients she can reach than those she cannot. And if she decides to treat them equally, even though she cannot connect emotionally with them all, then she must use one or more **general principle** (treat everyone equally or advocate for patients' interests, for example) – a method many nurse theorists reject.

As she investigates, Stephanie discovers that the tense atmosphere is partly caused by conflict between patients. The **Angry Man** is angry with the world, and is taking it out on the nearest target – the **Groaning Man**. Colleagues inform her that the **Sad Man** has become depressed by the pettiness of his fellow men, even as each faces profound illness. And the **Sleeping Man** has apparently taken sleeping tablets brought in by his wife, in order to escape the groans, moans and tears.

Knowing this, she sympathises with each of her patients. But feeling sorry for them is not enough. In order to improve the situation she has to decide who she should support first – should she calm the **Angry Man**, or should she console the **Sad Man**? Whatever she decides she will have to make a judgement – she must somehow discriminate between the four people.

But **the ethics of care** offers her no help. She has no framework to operate in, and no theory to stand on – and without these she and her patients are left vulnerable to capricious behaviour.

In fact, the situation in the four-bedded ward has been brought about partly because the consultant and two senior nurses have decided that the patients must stay in the same room, despite the **Angry Man**'s protests. It has also been caused by hospital policy (the room was originally intended for only two beds, but resource problems have forced a change) and by the consultant's disinterest in the feelings of his patients. He is concerned only that each recovers as quickly as possible from their surgical wounds. After that they are off his hands, either discharged or passed on to different specialists.

If she is to mitigate the effects of uncaring behaviour she needs more than involvement in patients' suffering. What she needs is a plan.

## SUMMARY

Nurse theorists advocate the **ethics of care** or **nursing ethics** as an antidote to an analytic approach that is often **tender-less**, and sometimes cruel. However, in their enthusiasm to compensate for the excesses of technological medicine, nurse theorists overreact. They correctly identify the inadequacies of the analytic method, but at the same time are blind both to its benefits and to the inadequacies of their own proposal.

### THE MAIN PROBLEMS WITH THE INTELLECTUAL APPROACH

1. It is contrived. Its language is only one of many possible languages in which to describe health care goals. Used in isolation, the intellectual approach creates a world in which only those things that can be readily measured are considered valuable. The more this world is favoured, the less visible the indefinable aspects of life become.
2. The intellectual approach can become so technical that it can appear not to be based on values. This effect is so strong that countless economists and policy-makers openly deny that they are biased – even though their work is quite obviously prejudiced when seen from outside their closed world.
3. It fosters a view – to which many clinicians are already inclined – that all human problems have technical solutions.

# THE MAIN DIFFICULTIES WITH NURSE THEORISTS' ALTERNATIVE

According to nurse separatists:

> ...the field of nursing ethics is now formally recognised, at many levels, as a discrete field of inquiry in its own right...[91]
>
> Nursing ethics today is a subject of study in its own right. It can no longer be regarded simply as a branch of medical ethics or ethics in general...[92]

However:

1. **Nursing ethics** (or **the ethics of care**) is inadequate to cope with most of the human problems nurses routinely encounter. In the hectic, pressurised settings of modern health care (where nurses come and go as shifts change, and patients find it difficult to know who is supposed to be looking after them) more is needed for creative, reliable decision-making.
2. The nurse theorist alternative is too reliant on each nurse's ethical intuition, and ability to empathise with all patients.
3. The caring approach has no problem-solving method to offer, and fails to clarify the meanings of its key terms.

In general, nurse theorists believe that:

> In pursuing the development of a substantive bioethic, nursing must reject the tradition of the destructive dichotomies that have dominated Western philosophical thought and scientific medicine...
> (There is an) urgent need for a radical new direction in moral thinking. The direction this moral thinking should take is clear. It must strive to:
> [...]
>> *construct a theory which is firmly based and shaped by practice, viz. The concrete circumstances of life;
>> *recognise the importance of shared lived experience, context, and the significance of interdependency...
>> *bridge the yawning gulf that has emerged between, for example, fact and value, objectivity and subjectivity...
>> *accept that there are some things that cannot be rationalised and objectively defined, and that some of our most decent human acts may be beyond rational explanation...
>
> Nurses are in an excellent position to contribute to the development of a substantive and integrated bioethic. All that remains...is for them actually to do it – and to do it competently and without delay.[29]

This would be a most welcome contribution, but it isn't going to happen spontaneously. Aversion to something is not enough to provide a better alternative. Even if it is correct to say that abstract principles divorced from practice and applied cold-heartedly to solve problems are bad and should be replaced, it is troubling that nurse radicals cannot say what they should be replaced with.

It is worse still that so many are struggling down such a clearly sign-posted blind alley. If ethics is a mysterious and intuitive process then it cannot be taught, and we do not need any more books or papers on nursing ethics. However, since not every nurse is able to empathise effortlessly with her patients, since not all patients want her to, and since there are some situations in which the intuitive approach is no help, there is more to say. We need to work out how to apply practical wisdom and tender insights to improve people's lives.

*SECTION TWO*

## CARING AND THINKING

Nurse theorists hope to find an ethical method that is nursing's own:

> ...a model for nursing ethics that is context-sensitive, rather than universal in nature, needs to be developed.[76]
> Nurses are in an excellent position to contribute to the development of a substantive and integrated bioethic. All that remains...is for them actually to do it...[29]

But since they disown intellectual analysis as part of:

> ...(a) tradition of...destructive dichotomies that have dominated Western philosophical thought and scientific medicine...[29]

they have no way forward.

To rebel against insensitive medicine by discarding the analytic method altogether is to lose too much that is good. Analysis is simply part of how we negotiate the world as human beings. It is employed by both men and women, professional and non-professional alike. There are better and worse forms of it, but some analysis is unavoidable if one is to proceed in a sane manner. If 'planning' means working out what goals to pursue and 'analysis' means working out how best to achieve them then we are all planners and analysts – even before we are able to crawl.

In order to achieve the most moral results, caring and thinking must be joined. They are not incompatible. Being sensitive to others' needs and thinking carefully about how best to meet them are not only complementary, they are necessary for decent practice. Occasionally just one or the other might be sufficient, but in the majority of cases both are required for practical moral reasoning.[93]

A few nurse writers have tried to point this out, bravely bucking the trend:

> ...neither moral principles and absolutes nor the ethics of natural caring can act as sufficient guidelines for a moral life or in decision-making. Instead these dimensions need to be considered together to deal with ethical dilemmas and possible solutions in any given situation.[94]

## THE CARING GRID

As they seek a feminine, non-universal, context-specific, caring ethics, many nurse theorists are hoping to break new ground. Yet such ways of ethical problem-solving

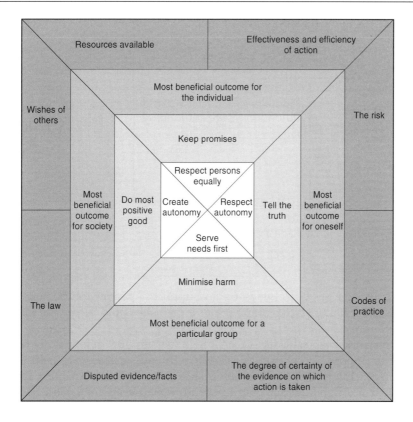

**Figure 8**   The Ethical Grid

already exist within the Western tradition.[95] One in particular – **the Ethical Grid**[15] – seems to be exactly what nurse theorists are looking for.

The Ethical Grid is a decision-making instrument sometimes employed in practice, though mainly used to help teach ethics to health workers of all kinds. It was derived from a theory of health – the **Foundations theory** – and is fully explained elsewhere.[15] Without an appreciation of the philosophy that underlies the Grid it is tempting to dismiss it as yet one more 'objective', 'mechanical', 'masculine', 'intellectualised', 'abstract-principled' monstrosity. Yet this is far from the truth.

The Ethical Grid is illustrated in **Figure 8.**

To use it one should reflect on a particular issue with reference to the boxes, and try to reach a decision based on one or more of them. An example of the Grid's use is given at the end of this chapter, as Stephanie solves her problem. However, for present purposes only the nature of the Grid need be explained.

## THE GRID'S NATURE

The Grid's central boxes, as normally depicted, are shown in **Figure 9**.

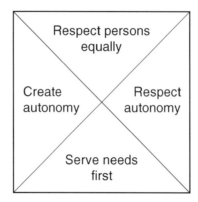

**Figure 9**   The central boxes of the Ethical Grid

These boxes mean:

1. The health worker should always try to support a person (or persons) in ways conducive to her being able to do or be more than she could before the intervention (**create autonomy**).
2. The health worker should try to enable a person (or persons) to become as autonomous as possible as soon as possible – intending always to help the person in question reach a point at which her wishes are paramount (**respect autonomy**).
3. The health worker should work on the central conditions for health before doing anything else (**serve needs first**).
4. The health worker should treat everyone equally unless there are compelling reasons why not (**respect people equally**).

It may be that these boxes look too confident and assured on paper. Possibly the Ethical Grid's squares and triangles convey a misleading impression of masculine precision. But once the philosophy behind it is properly understood the Grid can be seen for what it is – a serious way to treat other people considerately.

It is important to make this as clear as possible. It would be a tragedy if nursing were to reject the Grid's humanity forever, merely because of a misperception (an ideological bias caused by the **integrative tendency** – see **Chapter Five**).

## THE GRID IS NOT BASED ON THE ETHIC OF RIGHTS

Here's how Carol Gilligan characterises the **ethic of rights**, the foil to her **ethic of care**. The **ethic of rights** is:

a. A fair 'system of rules for resolving disputes'.
b. Respect or concern for 'the generalized other', not particular people.
c. Impartial.
d. Equally concerned for all individuals.
e. Based on the primacy of universal individual rights.

Whereas the **ethic of care** is to do with:

a. **Nurturing relationships with particular others to whom one is related in some way.**
b. **Solving problems within these relationships.**[77]

One can understand why even the Grid's central boxes might seem to be part of the **ethic of rights**. They do not mention particular individuals, they express the importance of treating people equally, they talk of the potential primacy of individual wishes, and they are supposed to be used to enable people to do or be more.

But on the other hand the Grid is clearly not a 'system of rules for resolving disputes', nor is it based on the primacy of universal individual rights, and nor are its boxes meant to be used impartially. Moreover, when seen in context even those notions that appear to be in keeping with the **ethic of rights** are not what they seem.

If anything, the Ethical Grid rests on a feminine understanding of the world.

## THE GRID IS FEMININE

The distinction between 'masculine' and 'feminine' is another 'destructive dichotomy' that ought to be avoided. However, despite its artificiality, I shall accept the terms temporarily in order to begin to elucidate the Grid's character.

I take 'a feminine approach to ethics' to be one that **intends to nurture, is concerned with relationships and connections between people, and is not based on rigid rules and inflexible principles**. If these qualities are feminine then the Grid is feminine because it identifies work for health as a thoughtful endeavour meant to strengthen other people's physical, social and emotional environments. To use the Grid well is to act like an intelligent, kindly mother to all those one can reach.

## THE GRID IS NON-UNIVERSAL

If 'universal' means based on 'objective moral truths', 'applicable in all social contexts', and 'of equal value in all cultures' then the Ethical Grid is *not* universal.

At a glance the Grid might seem nothing more than a set of commandments – you must respect individuals' autonomy, do no harm and so on – coupled with routine Western ethical dictums – maximise utility and obey the law, for example. But this is not so. Firstly, the central boxes apply only if one **decides** to work for health (See **Chapter Ten**). Secondly, each of the central boxes can be overridden by just one other central box, and in exceptional circumstances by non-central boxes too. Thirdly – and of most importance – the Grid is not a set of moral truths, it is merely a suggested framework to guide actions some people may consider moral in certain social contexts.

The Grid is not 'of equal value in all cultures' since not all cultures share its presuppositions. Indeed, some cultures reject outright the general Western understanding of ethics (which in any case consists of many different moral outlooks):

> For Hindu thought there is no Problem of Evil. The conventional, relative world is necessarily a world of opposites. Light is inconceivable apart from darkness; order is meaningless without disorder; and, likewise, up without down, sound without silence, pleasure without pain.[96]

> The association of the peace-loving doctrine of the Buddha with the military arts has always been a puzzle to the Buddhists of other schools. But one must face the fact that, in essence, the Buddhist experience is a liberation from conventions of every kind, including the moral conventions.[96]

Even within Western culture the Grid is not 'applicable in all social contexts'. It is meant to be used only in those situations where someone is expressly trying to improve the health of other people, and is useless in any other circumstances (in an adversarial legal process and many commercial situations, for instance).

Moreover, the very categories that make up the Ethical Grid are fluid and replaceable. For example, the Grid emphasises duties and consequences because it seems this is the way most of us deliberate – we ask 'should I . . .?' do this and 'what if . . .?' I were to do that. But these considerations could be replaced with alternatives, perhaps an emphasis on virtue – 'it is right that I do this . . .' – or intuition – 'I feel deeply that this is what I must do, though I can't fully explain it . . .'. And the central boxes might also be substituted, either by an alternative understanding of health[97] or by different categories of purpose altogether (the key points of socially responsible business practice, or pacifist politics, for example).

I doubt a theory could be more non-universal than this and still advance a positive moral position.


## THE GRID IS CONTEXT-SPECIFIC

Though it is possible to experiment with past cases or even hypothetical ones when learning to use the Ethical Grid, it can be brought into play in the practical world only if there is a concrete problem to be solved. It is quite impossible to use the Grid with reference only to Gilligan's 'generalized other'.


## THE GRID IS MEANT TO NURTURE

Most important of all, the central boxes are not hard-edged decrees. Rather they are supportive, nurturing ideals. In order to rectify any false view, the wording of the central boxes can be softened without loss of original intent.

For example:

**Create autonomy (1)**
**Respect autonomy (2)**
**Respect people equally (3)**
**Serve needs first (4)**

Might become:

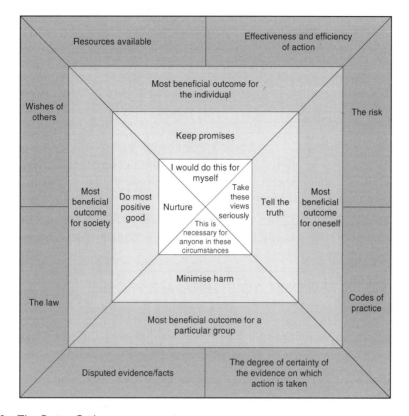

**Figure 10**   The Caring Grid

**I should nurture this person/these people (1)** (create autonomy)
**I should take this person's/these people's views as seriously as I take my own (2)**
(respect autonomy)
**I would do this for myself (3)** (respect people equally)
**This is necessary for anyone in these circumstances (4)** (serve needs first)

This gives a more explicitly caring Ethical Grid – see **Figure 10**.

This version is more cumbersome, but it ought now be easier to see that the Grid is none of the rather chill things it has sometimes been said to be.

It is not cold. It is meant to foster empathy. It is not objective, but based on a subjective sense of duty (originally my own) to respond to the needs of other people – both specific individuals and groups, and all of us in general. Nor is the Grid mechanical. There are several different ways of using it.[15]

In those cases where relationships are central then the Grid may carry its user to precisely the approach the **ethics of care** recommends. If autonomy is best created by exhibiting passion for a patient then the moral nurse should do this. If a group of people need unconditional support more than anything else then the nurse should give it, if she possibly can. If it is crucial to treat people unequally – if some people want relationships and others don't for instance – then the nurse can and probably should decide to do this. The only prerequisites are that the Grid is used to promote health[15] and is used with integrity. It is not even correct to call these requirements rules, they are looser than that. All that matters is that the ethical nurse should want to enhance other people's lives and will if appropriate give of herself to do so.

The Ethical Grid is neither intellectualised nor abstract-principled. It requires only average mental agility and research skills, all its central ideals stem from an argued **prejudice** for health, and (in my considerable experience) it is used as well – and in the same manner – by both sexes.

Though it was crafted by rational analysis – and could not have been invented without years of analytic training – the Ethical Grid is more to do with love than anything else. Unless you really care about what happens to other people you can never use it in the right way.

The following example of the Grid in use is meant to illustrate the above points.

## A CARING GRID RESPONSE TO STEPHANIE'S PROBLEM

After forming an initial impression of a situation, using any version of the Grid the user has to pose a specific question or spell out a hypothesis to test. The simpler the question or statement, the more effective the subsequent deliberation tends to be.

Here is a third way Stephanie's ethical exploration could have gone.

Reeling from the **Angry Man**'s outburst, Stephanie decides to examine the first hypothesis that occurs to her: **I should do what the Angry Man asks of me**. She withdraws from the room – promising to return as soon as she can. 'I need to think about what to do', she tells the **Angry Man** and the **Sad Man**. Then she goes and sits quietly in a side room. As a novice user of the Grid she begins her review at the outer layer – the level of practicality. She looks at all the boxes and tries to focus on the most relevant, homing in on the **risk, effectiveness and efficiency of action** and **resources available**.

What if she moves the **Groaning Man** out of the room? What if she increases his pain relief, as the **Angry Man** wants? In both cases she will run a big personal risk, since she has no authority to do either of these things. The least dangerous of the options would be to move him temporarily to an empty room (there is one available) – but then what would this achieve?

As far as Stephanie can see it would only be a temporary solution, and might well cause further problems. On the other hand, all other staff are fully stretched at the moment – Stephanie is the only resource available and cannot see how she could do much else.

Moving in a layer within the Grid, Stephanie wants to decide what her priority is. In particular she asks: am I concerned to achieve the most benefit for myself, for an individual, or for a group of people? She decides, almost instantly, that she should try to achieve the most beneficial outcome for all the patients – and for herself too, if possible.

Then – like the health economist, or indeed anyone else making any plan – she needs to decide what the **benefit** is in this case. Does she want to restore calm? Or should she select some other goal?

Because she is using the Grid Stephanie does not have to decide straightaway. She has two further layers to reflect on first, and these might help her arrive at a definition.

Still she addresses her hypothesis: **I should do what the Angry Man asks of me**. What are her obligations? **Telling the truth** and **keeping promises** don't seem directly important in this case – though **minimise harm** and **do most positive good** do. But again, to decide what 'harm' and 'good' are she must first decide what her basic goals are.

So she turns to the centre of the Grid:

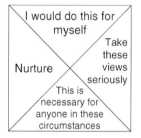

As she does so something important happens. She feels differently. It is only as she considers these four ideas that she begins to engage properly – personally – with the sufferers in front of her. Previously her analysis seemed more like an abstraction. It was as if she was searching for **the** right answer – the technical rule to sort out the problem, according to the tenets of professional nursing. But now, though no less difficult, everything is human.

She thinks about **each of the central phrases in turn**, testing out how it would be if she pushed the **Groaning Man's** bed out of the room:

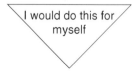

If I were the **Groaning Man** – and if I knew what was being done to me – I would hate it. I would feel shoved out, discarded – an irrelevance. And I would be furious about being singled out for something I couldn't help. I would not do this to myself.

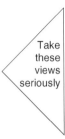

But what about this box? Stephanie thinks. Doesn't it mean I must respect the wishes of the **Angry Man**? He does have a point and I know I would want my views taken seriously were I in his position.

But – because she is analysing as well as empathising – she remembers she has already decided that her priority is the group as a whole, and as yet she knows only the **Angry Man**'s views. There are three other people to take into account.

Then, as she thinks '**Angry Man**', it jars her that she doesn't know anyone's name. She resolves to deal with this as soon as she gets back.

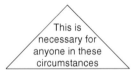

At the moment this notion seems less clear than the others. Stephanie recognises that in order to work out what is necessary for everyone she needs to discover more about the situation.

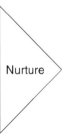

Thinking about this expression as deeply as she can – and noticing how much harder it is to want to nurture than to apply some hospital rule – she concludes that the approach she had in mind is fundamentally wrong. And she is shocked at herself.

She was wanting to solve an **irritating** problem as swiftly as possible – in order that she could move on and do something else. But what else would she do? It would either be a routine task (form-filling perhaps?) or would involve different patients. And then what would she be trying to achieve? Probably she'd be looking for a way out of the next situation so as to move on again – but what is the point of doing this? If there is any point to what I do – she thinks excitedly – it is right here right now.

'The very reason I wanted to become a nurse is to give strength to others, and yet all I was thinking was I want to get past this situation. I've had this wrong,' she realises.

Her task – she decides – is **not** to do what the moaning man tells her – it is to be a nurse and that means working to create a **better** situation – and to do so by supporting all the people in the room.

Now this isn't easy to do, but Stephanie knows some of the philosophy that underpins the Grid,[15] and decides to draw on it as best she can. She knows that working for health (the central boxes' inspiration) is much more than dispensing medicine and spouting hospital rules – and more than analysis too. She knows that to do it properly requires thinking about the key conditions – or foundations – needed by those she is seeking to help (not the foundations needed by just anybody, the foundations needed by these people in these circumstances in front of her at this instant).

She knows too that there are five central foundations she should think about (see **Chapter Eight** and **Figure 11**). In order to nurture, she needs to check out the state of each person's basic needs (1), what and how much each person knows (2), how much they understand and how they understand it (3), how they feel about the other people to whom they are related either by proximity, history, or emotion (4), and to correlate all this with their most prominent, present problems (5) (in this case, the reason each is in hospital). She also needs to check out the state of the foundations for any relevant **grouping** of people – so in this case she needs to think doubly hard. For example, she might ask: What does this group of people understand about itself? (1) Do they feel connected or not? (4) Do they have a **collective** crisis? (5).

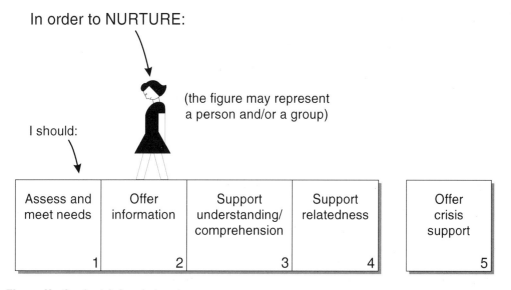

**Figure 11** Stephanie's foundation picture

## BACK IN THE ROOM

Stephanie has moved on. By thinking about the point of what she is doing she has ruled out what she now sees as a careless approach (to obey the loudest patient), and she returns to the room to take each of them seriously – as she puts it. In order to do this she acts spontaneously, with the four central boxes and their underpinnings constantly in mind.

She has decided that her task is basically **to nurture** in this situation, focusing on the 5 loose categories pictured in her head (and at **Figure 11**).

## WHAT DOES SHE DO?

She enters and goes to the bed of the **Angry Man**. She smiles at him and touches his shoulder.

'I'm sorry I went away. I needed a moment to think.'

'I'm Stephanie – and I'm a junior nurse. What's your name and what do you do when you're well?'

Still angry, but pleased and surprised to be treated as a normal person, the **Angry Man** replies:

'I'm Alan. And before I got this damn cancer I was an office manager.'

'In what industry?' she asks.

'Insurance. Life insurance', Alan laughs bitterly.

'Alan, you know when you were a manager – did you shout at your staff?'

'No, but that was different . . . they had to listen to me I guess.'

'And if you had shouted at them, what would they have thought of you?'

'OK Stephanie, I get your point – but what are you going to do for me? It is bad enough being ill, but here it feels like I'm being tortured. I've not only lost my health, I've lost my power. I've lost my identity. Do you know what I mean?'

It is a plea for help.

'I think I understand.'

**(She is taking him seriously and assessing his needs at this point.)**

The **Groaning Man** continues to groan, at times with distressing volume. Stephanie checks his vital signs, and his chart. There seems to be no cause for alarm.

'Do you know what his name is?'

'Brian, I think. He's only been here since yesterday. He's had some sort of stomach op. He's been crying like this ever since. Why don't the docs do something for him?'

'I don't know for sure. Though I am sure there's a reason. I'll ask as soon as possible and tell you what is going on. He certainly won't be like this for ever.'

'And until then I have to put up with it?'

'Well, you all have to put up with it. Him most of all, don't you think? And you can walk – why not go out for a while? Or use headphones?'

**(She is checking his sense of community – and isolation – and sowing seeds of compassion.)**

Alan looks at her blackly.

'I know', she says, 'but you do have options. You can come out and talk to me some more if you want?'

He nods.

'Can I? That would be nice. I might do that.' He lies back on his raised pillow, and shuts his eyes.

Stephanie moves over to the **Sad Man**, and attempts to engage him in conversation. At first it is as if he cannot hear, but after a few minutes he turns and looks at her. With the foundation picture (**Figure 11**) in her head she talks gently with him. She wants to find out how unhappy he is, whether he needs anything she or anyone else can offer, what he knows about his condition, what he knows about the other people.

'Has anyone introduced them to you?' she asks.

'Of course not!' he replies, astonished.

So she tells him their names and a little about what has happened to them. Does he know how that might feel? Can he relate his own pain to theirs? Does it help him understand why they are not behaving as he'd like them to? Does he think he could even help any of them?

He's not ready for that, but she has now at least examined two of the patients' foundations, and tried to enhance them a little in the process. She didn't calculate that she should approach these two before Brian, the **Groaning Man** – she just did it because it felt right. If she had discovered something significant about Brian – or if his medical condition had worsened – then she would have assisted him immediately, but that wasn't the case.

Stephanie resolves to come back to speak with the **Sleeping Man** when he wakes, to ask the doctor about pain relief for Brian, and then to discuss the situation with everyone, as a group, when all four can be part of the discussion. She sees that a large part of this problem is that each of them is in unnecessary isolation – even antagonism – with the others, and she can do something about this. She can nurture them together.

If she had to she could spell out these conclusions with reference to the Grid's boxes, but she doesn't feel the need, even though she has based her reasoning on them. Nor does she feel the need to relate her thinking explicitly to the underpinning foundations, though it is because she can see these boxes that she has been able to care so well. She is inexperienced and finds it hard to care intuitively – the philosophical ideas give her precisely the support she needs to enter the situation personally – and she is glad of all the help she can get to do her job the way she wants to.

If pressed Stephanie would say she used the boxes:
**respect people equally/I would do this for myself**
**create autonomy/I should nurture these people**
**maximise benefit for a particular group**
**effectiveness and efficiency of action**

But this would do her commitment an injustice. Her actions were both thought out and spontaneous, and it would be wrong to give credit only to those aspects of her work that can be named.

Sooner or later Stephanie – or perhaps a more senior nurse – may have to make a harder choice. Someone may have to suffer to benefit someone else. If Brian will not or cannot stop his loud moans then her tender approach may have to be balanced with some tougher reasoning. If so she will need to turn temporarily to a more clinical analysis, but she should never do so like the health economist – she should never do so without seeing the bigger, nurturing picture.

Only analysis can show when intuition is not enough. And only personal devotion to the point of one's work for health can show when reason becomes too ruthless.

# CHAPTER EIGHT

# Mental Health

## SUMMARY

This chapter:

1. Highlights disputed concepts in the understanding and treatment of **mental illness**.
2. Shows that nursing values cannot always be applied by nurses who work in mental illness institutions.
3. Extends the argument that it is time for nursing to:

    a. make its values theoretically and practically explicit;
    b. stand by these values and press collectively for change in those areas of mental health care where they do not currently apply.

4. Argues that if nurses are to nurse for mental health they need **an account of mental health** that coheres with a broad and practical understanding of work for health.
5. Offers, by means of a case study, a summary of the **foundations theory of health** and shows how this might be applied to promote mental health.

◆

## INTRODUCTION

For decades, academics and journalists have discussed the nature of mental illness, and what to do for or to those defined as mentally ill.[98] The debate continues to the present day, and shows no sign of abating (interested readers will find ample material on the subject in any library – for example[99,100]).

This chapter makes no attempt to contribute anything new to the discussion, but outlines two traditionally polarised positions – the **conventional psychiatric view** and the **anti-psychiatric view**. It is important that nurses are at least aware of this controversy, since their response will determine both how they deal with patients and how they might act to shape the future of mental health nursing.

Sometimes nursing ideals conflict with **the expectations of the mental health system** and sometimes – because of the nature of some patients' mental difficulties – **it is not sensible to pursue them**. In such circumstances, mental health nurses currently have no choice but to fall back on psychiatric understandings of mental health, even when they do not share them.

Nursing ought to strive to change this state of affairs.

## POLARISED VIEWS OF MENTAL ILLNESS

How nurses are able to nurse for mental health is presently determined more by the practice setting than by nursing philosophy. If the setting is dominated by pharmaceutical intervention, fear of danger, and staff anxiety, it is likely that the role of the mental health nurse will be to administer and monitor drugs, to keep order on the wards and to notify the psychiatrists of any troubling 'patient behaviour' – whether or not she thinks this is how best to create mental health.

But no independent-thinking health worker should be subject to context to this degree.

### AN EXTREME CASE

**Section One** discusses a rather extreme case in which a nurse might make a stark choice between participating in a regime attempting to **force a patient to change his behaviour**, and trying to **advocate for the patient** against the system.

Not all mental health care creates such alarming conceptual clashes. Neither are all mental difficulties addressed by drugs, even in the most chemically enthusiastic regimes. And nor is it always so difficult for nurses to empathise openly with their patients.[101] However, situations regularly occur in which opinions about how to work for mental health clash dramatically. These must be brought into the open so that nurses (and everyone else involved) can see the full range of conceptual and practical alternatives.

---

*CASE SIX*

### James and David – An Illustrative Conversation

James is a 35-year-old mental health nurse, David a 35-year-old patient on a compulsory treatment order, receiving psychiatric therapy against his wishes. David has a history of occasional violence against both men and women and has been to prison four times, twice for causing bodily harm and twice for theft.

David has also been a psychiatric in-patient three times – but not during the last three years. Since his twenty-first birthday David has been diagnosed with a variety of psychiatric illnesses, including **borderline personality disorder, schizotypal personality disorder, brief psychotic disorder** and **bipolar II disorder**.

*continues*

*continued*

He was about to be discharged from prison after completing his last sentence when the authorities had him assessed by two psychiatrists. The doctors agreed that David was suffering from a mental disorder and was a danger to himself and others. They reported 'a lack of insight', 'a history of non-compliance' and 'insufficient competence to make life-decisions'. They also wrote that newly developed drug therapies could eventually cure him, and would certainly alleviate his symptoms. They argued that David would be less likely to damage himself and others in a medium-secure unit.

In the three months since his admission – against which he protested furiously and articulately – David has received electro-convulsive therapy (**ECT**) for a 'depressive episode', anti-psychotic medication (**haloperidol**), has been kept in a locked ward and twice placed in seclusion for a week at a time (none of which he consented to).

James has assisted in the administration of both **ECT** and the anti-psychotic medication, and has no doubt he is doing the right thing. He thinks the matter is straightforward: David has a clearly diagnosed condition which is well-defined in authoritative textbooks and is treatable (currently his diagnosis is **borderline personality disorder** and **bipolar II disorder**). In James' opinion whatever it takes to cure David must be OK – whatever he says – since David is not in his right mind. Furthermore, James believes David has a right to this treatment – even though he does not want it – and society has a right to be protected from his recurring violence.

## QUESTIONS TO HIGHLIGHT THE CONCEPTUAL TENSIONS

Mental illness and mental health care is a philosophically elusive field. To help bring it into focus, it can be helpful to ask sharp questions:

1. Is David mentally ill?

2. Is David responsible for his actions?

3. Is David competent to make judgements?

4. If David is mentally ill, what are the chances he will be cured by his therapy?

5. What would a mentally healthy David be like?

6. How can I best help David become mentally healthy?

7. Is there anything I should not do to or for David?

The following section suggests answers a nurse like James might be expected to give to these questions. These answers are then challenged by an alternative voice (from the anti-psychiatric viewpoint) as if in conversation.

## A CONVERSATION BETWEEN DIFFERENT OUTLOOKS

### Is David Mentally Ill?

*James' Answer*

Yes. David has been diagnosed as having **borderline personality disorder (DSM IV 301.83)** and **bipolar II disorder (DSM IV 296.89)**. His records show that several experienced psychiatrists have previously concurred with these diagnoses. I could not question their judgements, and nor would I want to. David is obviously mentally ill.

*An Alternative Voice*

James, you have fallen for a myth. If you could read with an open mind the manual from which these diagnoses have been plucked you could not fail to see it for what it really is: the *Diagnostic and Statistical Manual of Mental Disorders* (edn IV)[102] (**DSM IV**) is a house of cards. Take away the raft of assumptions, see its axioms as hypotheses[103] and you are holding a speculative catalogue – one way of classification out of many alternatives. The **DSM IV** tries to fit people's experiences and behaviour into the sort of boxes found in other branches of medicine, in which pathological symptoms can be subjected to physical tests. But in the case of mental illness such tests do not exist – there are only behaviours and thoughts and psychiatrists' opinions about them.

Of course, drugs can affect how people feel and act. And some drugs can alleviate the symptoms of mental distress (they can lift depression and eliminate some hallucinations for instance). But this does not prove that mental illness exists in the way a broken leg exists.

Most drugs change how a person feels, and many alter how she thinks and behaves – anti-psychotics, alcohol, caffeine and adrenaline are each capable of doing this – but whether or not to describe **any** feelings and behaviours (however caused) as signs of illness is a human decision.

James, you cannot say that the behaviours you mention indicate **obvious** mental illness. Surely there is room for debate here. For example, David has had several different labels attached to him in his 'psychiatric career'. He now has two diagnoses – one of which refers to his personality (and there is nothing he or anyone else can do about this) – the other to a mostly depressive illness (and one might argue that it is reasonable for David to be depressed given his recent history). Given that he has already served his time for his criminal offences he should be given the benefit of the doubt and released forthwith. If he is violent again, caught and found guilty then he will have to take the consequences as laid down in law – end of story.

### Is David Responsible for His Actions?

*James' Answer*

Yes and no. A court found him guilty of stealing and violence and imprisoned him. At that time David was responsible for his actions and rightly held accountable by the law. However, his current behaviour is caused by his mental illness – which is a factor beyond his control – so he is not now responsible for the bad things he is doing.

The point where he starts and stops being responsible for what he does is not easy to specify. It may be that he is responsible for some of his actions – the trivial day-to-day behaviours, perhaps – and not responsible for others. But whatever the case, my role as a mental health nurse is not to worry about these theoretical matters but to treat David in line with the recommendations of the psychiatrists.

### An Alternative Voice

That isn't good enough. To justify treating David with drugs and electro-shock therapy you need to do more than this. What is he responsible for and what is he not responsible for? At what point in his prison sentence did his condition change to the extent that his status as a 'responsible citizen' changed? In what way is David's status different from 'mentally normal' people? To what extent are we 'normal ones' responsible for our actions? To what extent are you responsible for what you do? To what extent are you governed by your 'will' and to what extent is your 'will' under the control of your upbringing, your genes, your personality, your peers, your job, your anxieties, your ego? I bet you cannot answer, can you?

But if you cannot answer for yourself I do not see how you can possibly answer for someone else. Still less do I see how you can answer on behalf of someone who disagrees with you. David says he isn't ill and that he chooses to do what he does. He says he is sorry for his criminal offences, which he says he was provoked into. He says he has done his time and has a right to be released. If he offends again then that will be down to him – it is his responsibility. If he is caught he will take the blame and whatever punishment the courts lay down – but he will not be 'treated' for something he does not have.

## Is David Competent to Make Judgements?

### James' Answer

He is competent to make minor decisions for himself, like which TV programmes to watch (though even then I don't think he should watch violent or pornographic material). But he is not competent to make major decisions at the moment because he has a personality disorder, occasional delusions, and mood swings. What's more he lacks insight into his problems. So long as he thinks he is normal when he is not it would be wrong to allow him to make big social decisions for himself. He thinks people are plotting against him, sometimes he is very withdrawn and sometimes he has an elevated mood – these problems incapacitate his decision-making abilities.

Take his hunger strike, for example. This is not a sane judgement. It has been going on for four days now and if it continues his physical and mental condition will deteriorate further. For his own good, he should not be allowed to starve himself.

*An Alternative Voice*

You are confusing assumptions with facts again. You have decided to accept the opinions of the psychiatrists, but your choosing them does not make them true. David's behaviour has been labelled one thing by the Courts and another by medical people. That shows how arbitrary the labelling is.

The Courts said David did not make the right judgements when he broke the law, but was competent to make them. Now you say he isn't making the right judgements in hospital, therefore he is incompetent to make them. The only way David can be deemed OK by either of you is when he makes decisions you agree with (by abiding by the law in the first case and by acting according to the social values you favour in the second). Is this fair, do you think?

In fact I don't think the issue is about competence at all, for if David was consistently making judgements the system agreed with he would undoubtedly be regarded as competent to make them (and sane) – it is the judgements themselves that are the problem.

Given this I think all you can say is either that you don't like his actions and ideas, or that his brain is so damaged or impeded that he physically can't decide, or that his decisions are so inconsistent they make no sense.

## If David Is Mentally Ill, What Are the Chances He Will Be Cured By His Therapy?

*James' Answer*

There is a reasonable chance of success. And there is already good evidence that he is being made less distressed by his latest medication. He is much calmer and he now enjoys long periods of unbroken sleep (though there are some mild extra-pyramidal reactions at the moment).

David has not been physically violent since he arrived in the Unit. I'd say that the psychiatrists are doing a good job. I'm not saying his personality will change – or that he won't have problems with his thoughts and behaviours in future – but I do think we will eventually get David to the point where we can release him.

*An Alternative Voice*

What you are doing is wrong and what you are saying is mumbo-jumbo. It's a little complicated, so I need to separate some points out.

First, let's assume David really has an independently detectable mental disorder. Let's assume he is mentally ill in just the way his psychiatrists say. Now, in order to satisfactorily answer the question, 'What are the chances David will be cured by the treatments?' it is necessary to have evidence of the effect of these treatments on other people who have **the same diagnosis and are in roughly equivalent life stages and circumstances**. To do this we would need to undertake a specific research project – an experiment in which this particular therapy for this sort of patient is compared with other therapies (including non-psychiatric ones) and perhaps with no therapy. Since we cannot do this and since (as far as a literature search can uncover) no one else has done it we have to rely on the results of clinical trials of the drug haloperidol (brand name **Haldol**). We can't consider trials that compare haloperidol with non-chemical interventions, such as psycho-therapy, because there aren't any, as far as I can discover.

In the case of haloperidol used for psychoses I have discovered 841 publications[104] the great majority of which compare haloperidol with other therapies, but do not do so in a way that can indicate the chances of curing David specifically.

There are trials that involve haloperidol and placebos (146 papers)[104] – but these almost always involve other drugs as well.[105,106] Unfailingly, the research questions are – Is this drug better than this other one? or What is the effect of this drug compared to a placebo? – and never – Is this non-pharmaceutical approach better than the drug therapy marketed to psychiatrists?

Here is a typical example:

> Risperidone, a rather selective blocker of D-2 and 5-HT-2 receptors, was, in the doses 1 mg, 4 mg, 8 mg, 12 mg and 16 mg a day, compared to the rather selective D-2 blocker haloperidol in the dose of 10 mg a day, in 88 chronic schizophrenic patients. After one week placebo wash-out, the patients were randomly assigned to one of the six treatment groups and the study was performed as a double blind parallel-group study for 8 weeks. In the present analysis, a special emphasis has been laid on the effects on single symptoms and separate factors in the schizophrenic syndrome. Overall, risperidone in a dose of 4 mg a day was comparable to haloperidol in a dose of 10 mg a day. Risperidone was found to have a curvilinear dose–response curve with an optimum effect of 4 mg a day on the negative, anxious/depressive and cognitive factors and with an optimum effect of 8 mg a day on the positive and excited factors. While haloperidol had significant effects on the negative and anxious/depressive factors, risperidone had significant effects on all five factors – the positive, the negative, the excited, the anxious/depressive and the cognitive. The fact that the novel drug had significant effects on the cognitive factor might be of great importance as concerns the possibilities for rehabilitation of chronic schizophrenic patients.[107]

The existing research is, in my opinion, insufficient to make a meaningful judgement about the chances of curing David with haloperidol. No doubt you will disagree – but bear with me a little longer, for this is not my central argument.

Let's assume what I believe really is the case – that David isn't mentally ill at all. If this is so what are the chances of curing him, do you think?

Of course, he cannot be cured since he does not have a medical condition.

Let us look again at what is going on. There is no doubt that David **has** a problem and **is** a problem. The question is: (a) what problem(s) does he have (assuming for the sake of argument that he is not mentally ill) and (b) in what way(s) is he a problem himself?

I suggest his problems **are** these:

  i. He is being held against his will on the ground that he is mentally ill and a danger to others.

  ii. He is being sedated by a chemical which he does not want to ingest.

  iii. He is risking (involuntarily) a range of 'side-effects', some of which are known and some of which are only suspected.[104]

  iv. He is being coerced to behave in ways he does not wish.

He **is** a problem:

  i. Because his behaviours sometimes damage others.

  ii. Because members of the current system of social control (the courts, the gaols, the psychiatrists, the psychiatric institutions, the psychiatric nurses) have decided he is not fit to be free.

  iii. Because his treatment and detention is causing some debate amongst clinical staff, and this has tended to reinforce some people's attitudes against him.

Seen like this, the only way David can be cured is if he changes his way of behaving, and convinces the psychiatric authorities that he is no longer psychotic and no longer a danger to anyone else. The 'cure' is not the cure of an illness but an enforced change of attitude.

David has two choices. He can persist in his protests and assert his right to be released, or he can conform to the psychiatric regime and expectations (and bury his anger and resentments) in the hope this will be enough to get him off the compulsory order and back home.

## What Would a Mentally Healthy David Be Like?

### James' Answer

If David were mentally healthy he would not be violent and he would not be antisocial in other ways. He would realise his limitations and would want to work within these in order to be a useful member of society. He would not be depressed and he would not be so self-absorbed. David would recognise that not everyone likes him, but he would not suppose that this means that other people are out to damage him.

A mentally healthy David would be fulfilled and happy with his lot.

### An Alternative Voice

That is such nonsense. You are not talking about mental health but about what you think a satisfactory life is. You are conformist so you expect everyone else to be just like you.

We could disagree forever about what the good life is. However, what we do need to sort out – and which no one in mental health has yet managed to do – is **the philosophical basis for mental health work**. We need a practical theory of mental health in order to construct a general framework on which to base our specific judgements about what to do for the best in any given case.

# How Can I Best Help David Become Mentally Healthy?

*James' Answer*

By doing what I am doing. Our therapeutic work is removing his demons. This is the only possible way ahead for David – he is legally incarcerated and ours is the only therapy the legal system condones. No one and nothing else is going to be **allowed** to help David. Face it, there is no alternative.

*An Alternative Voice*

This is a very interesting question. Its answer is different dependent upon whether we are answering it with an ideal world in mind, or in the actual world only, as you are.

**In the Actual World**. As far as the actual world is concerned, this is an important question of strategy. Can the **caring nurse** operate effectively within a system which has concepts and goals in opposition to her own? If she can, what does she need in order to be successful (or at least as successful as she can be?).

There seem to be four strategies a nurse might adopt (combinations of them are obviously possible too). These are:

1. **To operate surreptitiously** – to support patients by talking to them quietly, explaining what is going on, outlining their options, trying to help them think clearly, trying to share whatever burden they have – while going along with the system and doing what is required by it (even if this is abhorrent to the nurse). Reason: it is better I'm here doing what I can than I'm not and someone else like James is.

2. **To refuse to go along with those aspects and practices of the system which do not fit with the philosophy of nursing the nurse espouses.** This refusal might take many forms, from outright rebellion and protest to reasoned refusal to join with selected practices (like **ECT**, for example).
At present it is unlikely that nursing organisations would support a nurse in actions of this sort.

3. **To go along with the system whilst working out, recommending and where possible implementing more caring practices** (allowing people to wear normal clothes, refusing to force medication on people, and so on).
A tough call, but possible if the nurse is articulate, focussed and above all stubborn.

4. **To refuse to go along with the system** whilst working out, recommending and where possible implementing more caring practices (allowing people to wear normal clothes, refusing to be violent and so on).
The chances are that were she to adopt this option, the nurse would soon lose her job.

To decide which of these will **create the highest degree of morality**[15] is not easy, and indeed it may be that whatever strategy the **caring nurse** adopts in the world as it is at the moment, it will make little or no difference – or will even be counter-productive.

**In a Better World**. In a better world health systems around the globe will have noticed the massive and sustained conceptual, scientific and ethical objections to psychiatry, and will have resolved to do something about them.[108] Health systems will – in a very much better world – have decided to start from scratch. They will ask not **'How can we improve psychiatric services?'** but **'How can we create mental health?'** And they would not automatically assume that psychiatry has **any** role in the creation of mental health, never mind a pivotal one.

In this very much better world mental health nurses would be regarded as important as anyone else, and their suggestions for change and policy would be taken seriously. If this world were to approach the ideal then nurses would have a well-worked-out philosophy of mental health – including practical definitions – and all sorts of ideas about how best to put it into practice.

## Is There Anything I Should Not Do To or For David?

*James' Answer*

I should not be gratuitously violent toward him. I should not be cruel. I should not use David to further my own ends.

*An Alternative Voice*

I agree with you. Unfortunately this is exactly what you are doing.

———————— ◆ ————————

The debate between **James** and the **Alternative Voice** is meant to illustrate that mental health nursing has to contend with ethical and conceptual problems no other branch of nursing has to face. However none of it is meant to be definitive – polarised positions are unlikely to be entirely right or wrong in a field as complex as mental illness.

There is everything to discuss, and yet psychiatric nurses are commonly expected to practise as if everything is known, agreed and fixed in stone. As a rule, nurses are supposed to take the word of a group of doctors, educated in little other than clinical technique and reductionist understandings of the world, that psychiatry is established to the same level of scientific certainty as surgery or haematology.

Psychiatry exerts such rigid control over so-called mental health systems that standard principles of nursing practice – even vaguely expressed – cannot always be applied in nursing work with people defined as mentally ill. If you are a mental health nurse, even if you think it is all right to go along with the system – and even if you believe there really is such a thing as mental illness and that psychiatrists and drug therapy are the way to deal with it – there will still come a point at which you will not be permitted to do what nurse theorists urge you to do in other areas of your work.

The **UKCC Handbook**[109] acknowledges this. It raises – but does not adequately resolve – central issues for nurse theory and mental health nursing practice. These form the subject of **Section Two** of this chapter.

# NURSE THEORY AND MENTAL HEALTH NURSING PRACTICE – A HEAD-ON CLASH

## THE PROBLEM THROUGH OFFICIAL EYES

The **UKCC 'Guidelines for mental health and learning disabilities nursing'** tries to highlight some of the tensions between nurse theory and the tasks of the mental health nurse.

The Guidelines explain that:

> There have been many changes in the way that clients are supported and cared for in recent years. Care has begun to move away from hospital settings and into a range of alternative settings. The particular needs of clients who require care in secure environments have been highlighted. Nurses working in all fields are often under additional pressure when making ethical decisions and the UKCC receives a great number of enquiries about the management of these dilemmas in the workplace.[109]

Understandably, the official Guidelines hold back from describing these dilemmas as what they really are: clashes of value and logic of fundamental importance for nurses and patients. However, fill in the missing reasoning and this conclusion is inescapable.

## EXAMPLE ONE: TO GET INVOLVED OR TO KEEP A DISTANCE?

For example, under the heading 'relationships' the Guidelines say:

> It is **your** responsibility as a registered nurse to maintain appropriate boundaries with clients. **If you are working with a vulnerable client, you must consider very carefully whether it is ever appropriate to have anything other than a purely professional relationship with the client.**[109]

This is surely sensible advice. However, contrast this with:

> One of the major constructs of [Watson's] theory is the transpersonal caring process. This process includes the notion of two phenomenal fields, defined as the totality of human experiences, coming together during an actual caring event … [both] nurse as giver of care and the client as receiver of care … being changed by the actual caring event. She defines this event as 'A focal point in space and time from which experience and perception are taking place …'. The intersubjectivity of phenomenal fields is characterized by both persons (nurse and client) being fully present in the moment and feeling a union with the other, a sharing of phenomenological fields.[110]

There is no denying that such moments happen in nursing, as elsewhere in human life. There is also no denying that moments of such intensity are memorably meaningful – and perhaps even give a fleeting glimpse of a deeper reality. However, there is an obvious and profound disparity between Watson's enthusiasm for the spiritual elements of nursing, and the UKCC's caution that:

> You must reflect very carefully before disclosing any personal information to your clients and should limit disclosure to that which has an explicit therapeutic justification.[109]

On the one hand there is the view that true caring involves disclosure of self by the nurse and an absolute sharing of 'phenomenal fields' by 'nurse and client'. On the other hand there is a clear and down-to-earth statement that mental health nurses should care only so far as they can justify on therapeutic grounds. If not:

> It may be necessary, following guidance from a supervisor, to withdraw from the care of a client...[109]

This is not a matter that can or should be glossed over. There are incompatible visions of nursing here. The one involves caring in an involved way for people whatever their difficulties and, by trying to understand those difficulties, gaining a deeper understanding of oneself. The other involves protecting clients and oneself by keeping a professional distance. It is impossible to have it both ways – so which one is real nursing?

## EXAMPLE TWO: MUTUALLY ACCEPTABLE OR IMPOSED SOLUTIONS?

Under the heading 'autonomy' the UKCC tries briefly to grapple with a central problem of health care ethics – to what extent is it acceptable to do things to other people in what you consider to be their interests but they don't? At paragraph 35 the UKCC says:

> You have a professional responsibility to promote client independence and autonomy. This means discussing with clients their proposed treatment or care. Decisions made by the inter-disciplinary team regarding the client's treatment or care should, where possible, involve the client and always be in the client's best interests.[109]

But of course unless 'where possible' and 'best interests' are explained the statement is of limitless meaning.[7] It is all very well to say that:

> You need to be able to make a professional judgement about the needs of clients by working closely with them to determine their priorities and identify mutually acceptable solutions to problems.[109]

But the ethos of contemporary mental illness systems is that mentally ill or intellectually impaired patients are not always in a position to identify 'mutually acceptable' solutions to problems. Mentally ill patients are generally not regarded as equal. Rather they are considered inadequate because their illness is thought (usually wrongly) to affect all their personal and intellectual abilities.[108]

The difficulty is made obvious under 'advocacy' in the UKCC Guideline. The booklet says (paras 29–31):

Advocacy is about promoting clients' rights to choose and empowering them to decide for themselves.

**Scenarios**

- You are asked by a client to support him in his appeal against detention under the relevant mental health act
- You are challenged by a carer for not understanding the needs of her son
- You become aware of a complaint by a client about his care

**Discussion**

You need to be clear about your role in advocating for clients. There is a potential for conflict when attempting to assume the role of an advocate, for example when patients are detained under the relevant mental health act. Your professional relationship with a client may mean that, because of your other responsibilities, it is difficult to be objective about your input and to identify and support the individual needs of the client. You must distinguish between your professional responsibility to advocate on a client's behalf and the role of a trained independent advocate . . .

When caring for groups of clients, you should establish whether they have particular needs which are not being addressed. This will include considering their physical, emotional, cultural and religious beliefs.[109]

These are difficult issues and no one can provide perfect solutions to them. However, nurses and 'clients' deserve a lot more directness – even honesty – from nursing authorities than this.

Let's place the Guidelines' advice in a typical 'mental illness' reality. What follows is part of an actual account – written by a mental health nurse and given to me – of the problems the system will not (seemingly cannot) face up to and change. What she says will come as no surprise to experienced mental health nurses.

In the nurse's opinion the Unit she works in is better than most, yet her report reveals a profound and systemic problem between nurses' aspiration to advocate (in either the normal or the nurse theorists' sense of advocacy) and the work they are employed to do.

# At the Unit

It seems to me that patients are relentlessly rendered powerless where I work. Here are some examples:

1. Those patients who are not confined to the Unit have to ask for weekend leave publicly, at a community meeting, and have to explain why they want it and what they intend to do with it. This would be difficult – embarrassing – even for people who are well and confident. Imagine standing in front of your office colleagues on a Thursday afternoon to ask permission to go to a seaside hotel with your new girlfriend – would you want to do that? For those who have mental difficulties it can be a source of great stress and anxiety – and could exacerbate certain conditions if patients feel they are being judged in some way. At the very least it is not a normal thing to have to do, and is not remotely empowering.
2. Decisions about who goes swimming are not made by the patients.
3. Discharge planning does not involve patients in consultation – plans are made for patients, not with them.
4. The Mental Health Act is rarely used positively. It is not available to patients and their rights under it are not explained. In fact it, and the threat of seclusion from other

patients, is often used as a threat: 'if you don't behave we'll place you on section X', 'the Act says we don't have to ask your permission . . .' and so on.

5. Patients who are not allowed to leave the Unit are made to dress in pyjamas. The only reason for this is to make it harder for them to escape, but its effects are to diminish the patients. They are made to feel different – almost a lower caste – they look strange, they are placed into a mode suitable only for patients hospitalised with serious physical sicknesses, they are regarded with suspicion by outsiders (it isn't normal to be dressed like this, so they must be crazy). In other words, the pyjamas are a burden and cannot conceivably be said to be of benefit to their wearers.

6. When patients want to see staff – including the nurses – they cannot summon them (like patients in hospitals for physical sickness), rather they have to knock at the central office and are forced to wait to be seen. It is hard to think of a closer analogy than a school child knocking at the staff room door, taking a chance that the teacher will see him.

7. Much of the language used by staff to describe patients is demeaning, and adds further to their being labelled and treated as children. A recent patient of mine (David) began as **borderline psychotic** and **personality disordered**, but as the months passed and he would not bow down to the psychiatric regime he became a 'management problem' – success in treating him was that he calmed down, became more compliant and less angry. Patients are not usually talked of as 'competent', 'bright', 'assertive' and 'well-organised' (unless they are about to leave, and not often then). Rather their behaviours (it is easier to deal with behaviours than complex human beings) are described as 'misbehaving', 'attention seeking', 'inappropriate' and so on.

8. Very little is explained – not even why a Unit is locked at one time and not another.

9. First names are used routinely for all patients, but not necessarily for all staff. While this has become acceptable amongst young people and those into their forties, people of older generations can find this uncomfortable and patronising – they expect to be called Mr or Mrs, and reserve first names for those few people with whom they are very close. To be called by a first name when you do not want to be can further undermine a patient's understanding of herself – and might even be said to be abusive.

None of these things are deliberate policies. They just happen. And in the absence of positive reasons to change them they continue and patients suffer in a place where nurses are supposed to be helping them.

There is impressive evidence from around the world[111–113] that partnership and co-operation work well in long-term rehabilitation and in the community – but the evidence is secondary in this matter. Since adults who are not defined as mentally ill welcome being treated with respect – and feel better when we are respected than when we are not – it is absurd and offensive not to treat mentally ill people with respect: you don't have to research this (and what research there is overwhelmingly supports this view[114]). Nurses who believe in patient dignity must advocate for these patients, or succumb to the system.

## EXAMPLE THREE: POLICE WORK OR HEALTH WORK?

In Western nations nurses are legally empowered to hold patients against their wishes. Section 5(4) of the UK Mental Health Act 1983 provides:

> If, in the case of a patient who is receiving treatment for a mental disorder as an in-patient in a hospital, it appears to a nurse of the prescribed class[(45)]

> a. that the patient is suffering from a mental disorder to such a degree that it is necessary for him to be immediately restrained from leaving the hospital; and
> b. that it is not practicable to secure the immediate attendance of a [doctor] for the purpose of furnishing a report under [section 5(2)],

the nurse may record that fact in writing; and in the event the patient may be detained in the hospital for a period of six hours from the time when the fact is so recorded or until the earlier arrival at the place where the patient is detained of a [doctor] having power to furnish a report under [section 5(2)].[115]

Whatever the rights and wrongs of forcible detention of people in mental crisis, it is clear that any nurse who invokes this power is not nursing in the **nurse theorist sense**. She is not 'being for the other' and nor is she 'offering information', 'helping a person find meaning in his illness', 'helping a person clarify what he wants to do' or 'doing things for a person that he cannot do himself'. Rather she is restricting, disempowering and controlling. For the time she is holding the person she is the police. No more, no less.

## How Can Nurses Be Advocates and Controllers?

Take the first situation identified by the UKCC:

> You are asked by a client to support him in his appeal against detention under the relevant mental health act.[109]

According to the **normal sense of advocacy** and the UKCC Code of Professional Conduct, Clause 1, which says:

> ... act always in such a manner as to promote and safeguard the interests of patients and clients

if your client asks you to support him against his involuntary detention then (at least according to this part of the UKCC's advice) you must advocate his interests. You should not advocate anyone else's interests. Rather you must:

> ... speak on behalf of some other person (or persons), as that person perceives his interests.

That's what **normal advocacy** is, but of course it is virtually impossible in reality for a nurse to do this, even in those cases where it is clear that an inmate is being wronged.[116]

## CAN THE MENTAL HEALTH NURSE ADVOCATE IN THE NURSE THEORIST SENSE?

Bring to mind Leah Curtin's belief that:

> ... the philosophical foundation and ideal of nursing is the nurse as advocate.[20]

There must be many thousands of nurses who think advocacy is what Curtin says it is. That:

> Explanations and working together with a patient are not extras that nurses may choose to do, they are the essence of nursing, the essence of the nurse–patient relationship.[20]

But is it likely in any of the circumstances described above? How, for instance, might the nurse advocate for David in the **nurse theorist sense** and at the same time continue to **be** a nurse in a medically dominated culture that sees people with mental difficulties as people to be coerced and manipulated into normal behaviours?[108]

## A FUNDAMENTAL CLASH OF VALUES

The UKCC Guidelines attempt the impossible – they try to reconcile incompatible outlooks on mental health care. Admittedly neither outlook is clearly stated (which is why the UKCC and other nursing bodies can get away with it for the moment) but it is clear enough that there are clashes in which it is possible to take only one side or another.

Simply compare the two outlooks:

---

### Nursing Priorities
The nurse is meant to do everything the Codes say. She is supposed to be respectful of all other people's beliefs, treat people as equals, care personally to the extent that she enters patients' subjective worlds, uphold their dignity, ensure their privacy, be ethical at all times, nurture all patients and – of course – work for their health (in this case work for their mental health).

---

### Psychiatric Priorities
The psychiatrist is trained to diagnose and treat mental illnesses supposedly as real and independent of the psychiatrist as cold sores and bronchitis.

---

The psychiatric system is modelled on the general medical system, in which nursing priorities are usually of secondary importance. In psychiatric work they can become irritations. If the goal is to remove symptoms and to change behaviours then the last thing the system wants is for its nursing members to reinforce patient attitudes by trying to understand their meaning.

## SUMMARY OF THE CLASHES

The chief problems for mental health nursing are:

1. **There are practical difficulties involved with entering into 'partnership' with people who are experiencing mental problems.**

    i. If the patient's view of life is badly distorted then how is the nurse to enter his world?
    ii. How can the nurse advocate (in the **normal sense**) the interests of the patient if the patient's interests are damaging to himself and/or to others?
    iii. How can she advocate in the **nurse theorist sense**? If she is supposed to provide basic needs for her mentally ill patient – and she thinks he has one set of needs and he thinks he has a different one – how can she possibly form the sort of partnership nurse theory requires?

2. **The role of the mental health nurse – at least in so far as involuntary detention and treatment are concerned – is to impede patients' freedoms.** Sometimes the impediments are locks, sometimes they are drugs to dull patients' thought processes, sometimes they are physical (holding them down to medicate them, or placing them in solitary confinement).

    The only possible justification for these impediments is that they lead to greater freedom for the patient in the long term. Whether these interventions actually produce long-term benefit is open to debate.

3. **The nurse has to work in a system which not only cannot satisfactorily define 'mental disorder'[117] but has no positive understanding of mental health.** Without such an understanding there can be no coherent way forward for the mental health nurse – negative notions (problems, illness, diseases, symptoms, distress) hold sway – eliminating them is everything (patients are commonly discharged without any attempt to create a more positive world for them).

## TIME FOR NURSING TO BITE THE BULLET

It is obvious from the amount of correspondence the UKCC receives on 'mental health' matters[109] and from the copious anti-psychiatric literature (much of it written by nurses and others with years of experience of the system[118]) that nurses frequently have to do things to patients (restrain them, drug them against their wishes, lock them up, control them, bully them, not take them seriously) that cannot possibly be justified according to the values favoured by the nurse theorists.

Nurse theorists and nursing bodies should stand up and say enough is enough – this is not what nursing work is about. This would not be to say that people with mental problems don't need help – nor would it be to say that sometimes people with mental health problems are not a danger to others (though the research shows they are far less dangerous than is generally supposed[119]). However, it would be to say that the present way of going about dealing with people labelled mentally ill is a conceptual, ethical and practical failure – and it would also be to recommend the many alternatives based on creative notions of health rather than restrictive notions of abnormality, dangerousness and safety.

There are lots of reasons why nursing does not do this. One of them is that nursing – like medicine – does not have a clear understanding of mental health.

**Section Three** of this chapter shows what is required in order to begin to make nurse theorists' tentative aspirations reality in mental health work.

*SECTION THREE*

## MENTAL HEALTH PROMOTION: A WAY FORWARD

*CASE SEVEN*

### A Case of Mistaken Identity?

22-year-old Peter Murray is from a family which has ancestral roots in a Scottish hamlet and the **Ngati Whatua** tribe of **Aotearoa**. The family can pass as pure Caucasian and live as European New Zealanders.

Peter is several kilos overweight. He has a criminal record for petty theft and joyriding, and was a notorious 'tagger' as a teenager (he used spray paint to leave an elaborate personal mark – or tag – on walls in public places).

Peter detested school and has no formal qualifications. He worked as a labourer for a while, but has been unemployed for the last eighteen months.

Peter has a handful of mates – almost all of Maori or Pacific Island descent – but is unable to talk with them at any depth. They crack juvenile jokes, smoke cannabis, grouse about *pakeha* (foreigners or Europeans), but they never discuss their dreary lives.

When alone – which he is most of the time these days – Peter feels sad to his bones. He cannot see how life can get better, and finds solace in pink-iced buns, alcohol and tobacco. He's recently slumped into watching TV all night, then sleeping most of the day. His mates have grown bored with him now he can't be bothered to come out stealing any more.

Last night, after watching **Once Were Warriors** (a brutally realistic dramatisation of urban Maori life) he slugged whisky until his throat went numb. Then he gently donned a Maori skirt, seized a broom handle and bolted from his flat.

Running quick and hard through dark streets he felt the wrath of ancestors pulsing through him, filling him with unearthly elation. Flying wild-faced through a deserted mall he boomed a *haka*, then stopped abruptly, half-squatting before High Street Electricals.

*continues*

— *continued* —

The broken handle, rock-steady in outstretched hands, cast a shadowy line beneath his fierce eyes. The stillness was intense. Yet he sprang at the window. One foot forward *kung fu* style smashed the heavy pane. Blood pumping onto shattered glass, screaming and whooping in a cacophony of joyous destruction, he attacked TVs as if they were wild beasts.

The police arrived, tyres and sirens adding their squeals to his. Three officers hurled him from the shop, over the pavement, into a filthy puddle by the side of the road. They cuffed his hands behind his back, then bundled him into a waiting ambulance, where he was sedated despite his kicks and curses.

Blue lights glaring they raced to the hospital. His wounds were stitched, then he was left on a single seat in a bare locked room, awaiting the psychiatrist. Peter had no idea where he was. Nothing made sense. As tears ran all he could think was . . . too far away . . . too far away . . . too far from home . . .

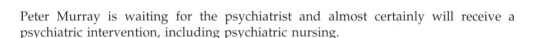

Peter Murray is waiting for the psychiatrist and almost certainly will receive a psychiatric intervention, including psychiatric nursing.

But does he need anything more? Does he need mental health promotion? Could nurses become mental health promoters? And what would this mean? In order to decide, any would-be mental health promoter (nurse or otherwise) must answer three **central questions**:

1. **What is mental health?**
2. **How, if at all, can mental health be promoted in these circumstances?**
3. **Will the health promotion strategy be ethically sound?**

Whatever the situation – whether it is Peter's crisis, the mundane routine of a wealthy white family, a pre-school classroom, or a community psychiatric nurse's workload – if mental health promotion is to be theoretically coherent, practically useful and socially responsible these questions are inescapable.

## WHAT IS MENTAL HEALTH?

There is no question more basic to mental health work, yet it is hardly ever properly analysed by aspiring mental health promoters (psychiatrists and psychiatric nurses included). Instead, either it is assumed that **mental health is something everyone understands intuitively**; or that **mental health is the opposite of mental illness**; or **mental health is said to be 'mental well-being', 'happiness', 'positive mental capacity'**; or the **various ideas are obscurely and uneasily combined**.

Two of these propositions dominate the current scene.

## THE MENTAL ILLNESS THEORY OF MENTAL HEALTH

Western health planners take it as read that mental health services should strive to ameliorate symptoms of mental illness. If they are called on to defend this assumption, advocates of the **mental illness theory** tend to make the following claim: symptoms of mental illness are abnormal, and of a form that can be found in any culture. Remove these symptoms and one is left with a normal mental state. This must be a mentally healthy state because most people are not mentally ill.[120]

This view has substantial **deficiencies**:

### i. The assumption that clinically defined symptoms of mental illness are the only indicators of a person's mental health

Reflection on Peter's situation quickly exposes the **mental illness theory's** shortcomings. The assumption that mental illness symptoms are the **only** indicators of mental health is strikingly inadequate. Even if it could be shown that Peter's outburst was caused by an abnormal chemical change in his brain[108] it makes no sense to say he had complete mental health before he became mentally ill.

Peter's health is weak because he is in no position to flourish – he has little or no chance of realising his enhancing potentials.[121] In fact he doesn't think he has any. Even if psychiatry can medicate away his 'delusion' or 'depression' Peter will still be an unemployed, miserable, frustrated, socially inept young man living in a society where most people have hope. He will remain a bewildered soul with no idea whether he is Maori or *pakeha*, and no inkling why it might matter profoundly that he decides one way or the other.

To understand even a little of Peter's life is to recognise **the absurdity of equating lack of symptoms with mental health**. It is obviously possible not to have symptoms of mental illness as defined by psychiatry and nevertheless to be heartbroken, ignorant, dull, unstimulated and unfulfilled. And it is equally possible to have symptoms of mental illness removed or subdued at the cost of brightness, feeling alive, feeling a sense of purpose, and feeling a sense of self.[108,122]

### ii. The assumption that mental health is normal and mental illness is abnormal

There is more than one sense of **normal**.

Peter is **statistically abnormal** since most New Zealanders (of any origin) do not experience the intense feelings and behave in the way he did. However, just because a person experiences statistically abnormal elation and behaves unusually relative to the rest of the population, it does not automatically follow that he is mentally ill.

If Peter had won Lotto (the NZ national lottery) he would have been abnormal in a comparable way. He would have been intensely happy, he may have run wild in the streets, he may have felt blessed, or lucky, or believed his ancestors were smiling on him. If so, it is unlikely he would be considered mentally ill. Although such a reaction would be **statistically abnormal** it would almost certainly be considered **understandable** – statistical abnormality does not automatically render a person mentally ill.

**Normal** used to mean **being understandable** has the effect of **equating mental health with behaviours and thoughts considered acceptable in a society** (so one might expect a liberal society to have a broader notion of mental health than a conservative one).

In a conservative system, for example, if a psychiatrist does not imaginatively attempt to comprehend a person's behaviour **for that particular person in those particular circumstances** then it is probable that **statistical abnormality** will also be seen as **not understandable**. In Peter's case, his behaviour is superficially inexplicable – the only explanation seems to be that he is insane. Why did he dress in that weird way? What did he think he was doing with the broom handle? What reason could there be for his crazy attack on the TVs? How could he not notice his serious injuries unless he was deranged? He said he heard his ancestors' voices – is this not a clear case of auditory hallucination?

But if you had seen *Once Were Warriors*, and if you knew Peter had been watching it that evening, and if you could think his resentful thoughts about the *pakeha* invaders, and if you could feel his guilt about his own family's part in that invasion, and if you had sat in front of the TV for endless nights, watching twenty minutes of adverts in every hour telling you to buy everything when you can afford nothing – then you might at least think twice before describing Peter's reaction as incomprehensible.

## THE WELL-BEING THEORY OF MENTAL HEALTH

This theory is just what it says – you are mentally healthy if you have well-being. However, its theoretical and moral weaknesses make it very difficult to defend as a basis for practical mental health promotion.

The **well-being theorist** has three alternatives. He can:

a. keep the notion of mental well-being ambiguous (which is what most writing on the **well-being theory of mental health promotion** does);
b. define it specifically; or
c. permit subjects to define it for themselves.

Each of these options has significant difficulties. If he keeps the notion vague it is hard to see how he can consistently recommend any practical health promotion strategy for Peter. If he defines mental well-being specifically then he is plainly making assertions of value, and will inevitably make practical recommendations of the type: Peter **should**, the government **should**, Peter's family **should**, and so on.[123] For example, he may say that a key aspect of mental well-being is to have supportive friends and meaningful relationships – an opinion held by many people of course, but not one which everyone shares. The more precisely the mental health promoter specifies the nature of these relationships the more chance the recipient will disagree (Can meaningful relationships exist only between people who are equal? Can and should they occur between commander and commanded? Should Peter shun his present mates? Should the mental health promoter seek to foster meaningful relationships only between Peter and radical Maori? Should the health promoter try to provide an environment – in an institution? – where completely new relationships can flourish?).

If the health promoter lets Peter define mental health for himself there is the obvious risk that he will specify it in a way the mental health promoter will be unable to accept. Peter might prefer to be left alone, for instance, while the health promoter believes this is the last thing he needs. Or he might decide to become militant, while the health promoter is convinced that the only way forward is to encourage bi-culturalism.

The **mental illness health promoter** at least has some non-subjective indicators to consider (a patient's agitation, specific symptoms, dangerousness) and knows that when these factors have been dealt with his intervention must cease. The **well-being mental health promoter**, on the other hand, has only his or the subject's view of well-being and in theory may continue to intervene indefinitely: which is a deeply ethically troubling prospect.[15]

# A BETTER WAY

There is a better alternative, known as the **foundations theory of health**. In the following section the theory is briefly explained, after which it is applied to Peter's case.

## THE BONES OF THE FOUNDATIONS THEORY OF HEALTH

The **foundations theory of health** has been developing for well over a decade, forms a large part of three books,[15,121,124] and cannot be adequately explained in a book chapter. Therefore in what follows I restrict my discussion to a short general outline of the basis of the theory, a brief synopsis of the theory's usefulness for health workers who wish to work for health with individuals and small groups, and an account of how the **foundations theory** might be applied to help Peter.

The **foundations theory of health** is derived from conceptual analysis of the meaning of health, from study of other theories of health, from empirical observation of work actually done in the name of health, and from certain untestable beliefs about the morality of social arrangements. My analysis of these matters has led me to conclude that any plausible account of health must understand the purpose of health work to be the identification, and if possible removal, of obstacles to worthwhile (or **enhancing**)[121] human potentials. That is:

> Work for health is essentially *enabling*. It is a question of providing the appropriate foundations to enable the achievement of personal and group potentials. Health in its different degrees is created by removing obstacles and by providing the basic means by which biological and chosen goals can be achieved.

> *A person's (optimum) state of health is equivalent to the state of the set of conditions which fulfil or enable a person to work to fulfil his or her realistic chosen and biological potentials. Some of these conditions are of the highest importance for all people. Others are variable dependent upon individual abilities and circumstances.*

The extent to which a person can function successfully (i.e. the extent to which a person is autonomous) is roughly the extent of his or her health

A person is enabled by the foundations to achieve chosen and biological potentials: if the foundations are complete - in context for the person - then he or she might be said to have optimum health

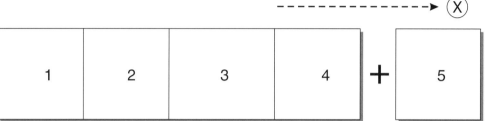

If the person begins to move towards, arrives at, or is driven towards (X), then additional provision or maintenance of the stage might be necessary

**Figure 12** An abstract depiction of health

The actual degree of health that a person has at a particular time depends upon the degree to which these conditions are realised in practice.[121] (Quotation slightly changed from original.)

This idea can be depicted in the abstract, see **Figure 12**.

The boxes in Figure 12 may be described either as **conditions for** health or **constituents of** health (though ultimately only the latter understanding can be sustained). Their importance, whichever way you look at them, is that they provide a platform for action. If a person can stand upon the four central blocks in good order then she will have a high level of health. If her boxes are in bad shape she will tend to have fewer options for fulfilling life performance than if they were sound.

How many different sorts of boxes there are, their exact content, and how important each is compared to the others is contestable, varies according to circumstance, and is at least partly a matter of human social judgement. On the foundations theory of health the numbered blocks shown in **Figure 12** have the following substance:

Some of the foundations which make up health are of the highest importance for all people. These are:

1. The basic needs of food, drink, shelter, warmth and purpose in life.

2. Access to the widest possible information about all factors which have an influence on a person's life.

3. The skill and confidence to assimilate this information. In most societies literacy and numeracy are needed in older children and adults. People need to be able to

understand how the information applies to them, and to be able to make reasoned decisions about what action to take in the light of their information.

4. The recognition that an individual is never totally isolated from other people and the external world. People are complex wholes who cannot be fully understood separated from the influence of their environment, which is itself a whole of which they are a part. People are not like marbles packed in boxes, where they are a community only because of their forced proximity. People are part of their whole surroundings, like cells in a single body. This fact compels the recognition that a person should not strive to fulfil personal potentials which will undermine the basic foundations for achievement of other people. In short, an essential condition for health in human beings who are aware of the implications of their actions is that they have an awareness of a basic duty they have because they are people in a community.

Other foundations for achievement are bound to vary between individuals dependent upon which potentials can realistically be achieved. For instance, a diseased person, a person in a damp and dilapidated house, a person in prison, a fit young athlete, a terminal patient, and an expectant mother all need the central conditions which constitute part of their healths, but in addition they require other specific foundations in order to enable them to make the most of their present lives.[121]

The idea is that boxes 1–4 represent the central conditions for a fulfilling life, and that lack of (or serious defect in) them will severely impede a person in the achievement of enhancing potentials. Box 5 represents additional support made necessary by individual circumstance. When faced with a life crisis people sometimes find that the four central boxes, even in excellent condition, are of much less use than usual. If people are 'falling over the edge' of their platform they will need the support of a fifth box. That is, they will require the:

> ...other specific foundations [necessary] to enable them to make the most of their present lives...[121]

The content of box 5 depends entirely upon the nature of the particular problem. Thus the fifth box may represent medical services and support; improved facilities for a disabled person; hospice care for a terminally ill man; special protection and counselling for a battered woman, and so on. The fifth box is needed when a particular life problem becomes bad enough to impede significantly a person's movement on the platform formed by the other four boxes. This box then either permanently extends the platform, substitutes for an irreparably damaged central box, or is the means by which a person is enabled to climb back onto her normal platform.

It will be immediately obvious that this notion of health does not have traditional medical provision as its focus. This is not a problem or an error, rather it is a logical consequence of the fact that work for health seeks to remove impediment to human achievement, and that problems that are tackled by medicine do not constitute a special category of impediment.[124] Just as a person becomes substantially immobilised in his life in general if he becomes seriously diseased or injured, so he is equally likely to be severely impeded in life if he does not have a home, or possesses no useful information, or has not been educated, or does not realise the extent to which he is formed by and depends on the existence of a community of others.

It may also appear that this theory of health implies that **any** effort to help people live better lives is work for health. However, while the theory certainly does extend the idea of health beyond medical endeavour, it nevertheless sets **limits** on the interests of health workers. The task for any genuine health worker working with an individual or a small group is to recognise the importance of the foundations in context – to identify with or for each individual those components which are lacking, or those which are most in need of renovation – and then to work on those aspects most appropriate to the skills of that health worker. In this way the theory begins to offer guidance to individual health workers, and may help establish practical priorities.

Crucially:

> . . . work for health cannot be fully comprehensive – not all work should be thought to be health work. Such a state of affairs is not possible, nor is it desirable to have professional interference in the name of health covering all aspects of individuals' lives. *Once suitable background conditions have been created, the achievement of the particular potentials that have been chosen is up to the individual and not the concern of health workers, although permanent maintenance work will often need to be carried out on the foundations.*
>
> The analogy of work for health is very close to the work needed to lay the foundations of a building. *Obstacles such as poor drainage, subsidence, awkward outcrops of rock (analogy: disease, illness, poor housing, unjustified discrimination, unemployment) have to be eliminated or overcome in some other way. Then firm foundations and reinforcements have to be added (analogy: good general education, confidence in thinking things through personally rather than relying on what one has been told, good opportunities for self-development). But, unlike the case of building construction, work for health should stop here.* What a person makes of the foundations he has is up to that person, as long as he possesses at least the essentials of the central conditions. Given this then an individual must be allowed to become the architect of her own destiny.[121] (Quotation slightly changed from the original.)

This understanding of health can be fleshed out – see **Figure 13**. This is a general elucidation only. In fact in every case – whether the figure represents a person, group or larger community still – the specific content will vary dependent upon the figure's circumstances. One way to imagine this is to think of a one-armed bandit – or the departures board at a large airport. When the matchstick figure changes so too does the content of the foundations – different concerns click into place dependent upon the prevailing situation.

A family who have a badly handicapped neonate, a 40-year-old with inoperable cancer and two young children, the increasingly forgetful septuagenarian – each will require the best foundations possible, but the exact nature, size and strength of each foundation will be different in each case. For example, the family with the handicapped neonate will require all five foundations in depth, and may particularly need boxes 4 and 5. In this case box 4 might be spelt out to mean all those supports already included in **Figure 13** plus extended contact with other families in similar situations. Box 5 will change from **Figure 13** and will reflect the specific needs of the baby (for medication, physiotherapy and so on) and the rest of the family (for counselling, grief support, extra financial support and so on).

Note that the **foundations theory** makes no distinction between obstacles that are primarily tangible (lack of painkilling medicine, lack of money) and those that are primarily mental (the family's lack of understanding of their situation, a sense of loss, confusion about how to carry on). There is no need to divide these obstacles into

| 1 | 2 | 3 | 4 | 5 ADDITIONAL OR CRISIS SUPPORT |
|---|---|---|---|---|
| A home to call her own for everyone in a particular society | Open access to the widest possible information | Education to good levels of literacy and numeracy | The constant awareness of one's belonging to a community – the awareness of the interests of others and of one's dependence upon others' thoughts, on their physical and cultural support, and on their productivity | Access to life-saving and sustaining medical services |
| Protection from death, assault, and undue coercion / Adequate daily nutrition | Assistance with the interpretation of information (e.g. legal, medical, technical, bureaucratic) | Education to enable a good level of unsupported interpretation of information | | Access to medical services that enable the restoration of normal function for the individual (ideally to restore the person to the full platform, left) |
| Assistance, whenever required, with defining and (in some circumstances) pursuing purposes/life plans | Encouragement to find, to explore, retain and act on information | Open, continuing education without bar of age | A constant awareness of one's duty to develop oneself and to support others – and so to develop the community | Access to special context-dependent support in medical crises |
| Meaningful, fulfilling employment | Encouragement of open discussion of information (public seminars, sponsored 'open info' sessions, public service talkback radio and television) | Encouragement of self-education throughout life | The constant understanding that citizenship involves not only individual fulfilment but a commitment to the larger civic (global) body | The continuing fulfilment of special needs – the absence of which would constitute crisis |

**Figure 13** The foundations with more specific content

separate categories for they are inextricably related: they are all part of the general problem. Attention to physical matters will have mental effects, and *vice versa*.

## THE FOUNDATIONS THEORY APPLIED TO HELP PETER

The **foundations health promoter**, faced with Peter distraught in his cell, has a daunting task. Indeed the task is all the more formidable because the **foundations theory** so plainly shows how much there is to be done.

The first challenge for the **foundations health promoter** is to assess Peter's situation (both in the present and more generally) with the theory fully in mind. In other words the **foundations health promoter** must thoroughly examine Peter's foundations to see how things stand. Only once everything is in the open is lasting progress likely.

At the moment it is unlikely – and in many institutional settings inconceivable – that **the mental health nurse** will be in a position to promote Peter's health in line with the foundations theory (it is almost equally unlikely that medically qualified workers will be any better placed). However, it is up to those who espouse nursing values to find ways to implement better practice – and to try to work according to an explicitly moral theory of mental health practice may be one way forward.

Notice, for example, that unlike the **mental illness theory** the **foundations approach** is not exclusively concerned with the question: **Is Peter mentally ill?** In fact this may not be a primary consideration at all. Unless there is an emergency the **mental health promoting nurse** will look first at boxes 1–4, and decide if there is a need for additional support after reviewing these.

There is insufficient room to conduct an extensive analysis of Peter's health needs – but it is important to explain enough to show that it makes no sense to focus on his mental life while ignoring everything else. In order to possess a reasonable degree of health (or ability to function on an adequate stage) Peter needs:

---

*BOX 1*

**At the moment:**
Immediate protection from hasty and potentially damaging health interventions
Rest
Fruit juice, and good food if he gets hungry
A friend or sympathetic person to talk to
A dependable solicitor

**Generally:**
A place that feels like home
Better nutrition
A sense that his life has a point
Fulfilling employment
Exercise
Ways to combat frustration and despair

---

---

### *BOX 2*

**At the moment:**
To know where he is
To know his legal rights
Suggestions about how to cope with this situation

**Generally:**
Information about alternative lives – both those that Peter himself might live and those others have lived (he needs information about educational opportunities, about careers, about history, about Scottish culture, about Maori culture)

---

### *BOX 3*

**At the moment:**
Help in understanding his rights
Help in working out what to do for the best

**Generally:**
Continuing encouragement to get educated
Education in **Te Reo Maori** (Maori language)
Education in Maori culture
Education in the history of colonisation

---

### *BOX 4*

**At the moment:**
To know that he is not alone
To know that other people have his best interests at heart
To know that other people are facing similar troubles

**Generally:**
Help in identifying the community to which he belongs, and then support in entering and participating in it

---

At the moment Peter's stage is incomplete, and almost all the pieces that do exist are in bad condition. There is crisis – and a very long way to go to get the stage right (indeed, to do so completely is beyond the skills and resources of any organisation other than the State). It may indeed be that Peter needs **Box 5** now – though it is not obvious what specific support should be offered from it. Perhaps medication will help. Perhaps it will be good for him to be treated in a mental hospital. Perhaps it will not. The **health promoting nurse** (if she has any influence at this point) will need to assess the evidence and the alternatives, and then do what she can to get him through this.

Critically, whatever additional support is recommended it must (a) **be most likely to restore Peter to his general stage as soon as possible** and (b) **be explicitly acknowledged to be a means toward this** (not an end in itself, or primarily a means of controlling him, or primarily a means of eliminating danger – this is the way to reduce autonomy, not to create it).

There should also be the most careful interplay between the **health promoting nurse** and Peter. It is possible his behaviour was prompted by a feeling of alienation – and by an inexpressible anger at the colonisation and exploitation of the Maori people. Given this the last thing the nurse should do is to set out to promote Peter's health with a clear end in mind – with a distinct mental picture of a healthy Peter two or three years from now. Any health promoter must constantly be on guard to do only those things which present Peter with the widest range of opportunities – which includes his choosing to live as a Maori, even as a Maori radical if that is what he decides. Unlike practices based on the **mental illness theory** and the **well-being theory of mental health** the **foundations health promoter** works directly on the platform, not the person's mind.

# SUMMARY: HOW DOES THE FOUNDATIONS THEORY ANSWER THE THREE QUESTIONS?

## WHAT IS MENTAL HEALTH?

Mental health is a part of the foundations which make up a person's health in general. Sometimes it may make sense to focus solely on a person's mental life, but usually it does not since we are at once physical, mental and social beings.

According to the **foundations understanding of health**:

> Health in general is created by removing obstacles and providing basic conditions in order to help individuals and groups achieve desirable and realistic chosen and biological potentials. **Mental health promotion is** a multi-faceted endeavour which works with people and on their environments to foster the achievement or maintenance of the mental strengths people need to deal successfully with life's problems. The prevention and cure of mental disorder may be part of mental health promotion, but is not necessarily a priority.

## HOW CAN MENTAL HEALTH BE PROMOTED?

By a theory of health that regards work for health to be the thoughtful removal of obstacles in the way of fulfilling biological and chosen human potentials, and by doing anything that can reinforce the foundations. This may include medical therapy, though sometimes medical therapy should be shunned by the health promoter, especially if it appears that it may damage existing foundations.

## ARE THE PROPOSED HEALTH PROMOTION MEASURES ETHICALLY SOUND?

Of the three theories of mental health promotion discussed in this section only the **foundations theory** has ethical limits built in. The point of the **foundations understanding** is to promote the autonomy of the figure on the platform, as effectively and speedily as possible, so that the figure itself can then decide how best to proceed. In other words the **foundations theory** has an integral safeguard against ethical stupidity and imperialism – it is a self-limiting theory of health work.

## MENTAL HEALTH PROMOTION SHOULD NOT BE A SEPARATE TASK

The **foundations theory** has some unconventional theoretical and practical implications for mental health nursing – but is all the stronger for this. In particular it asserts that **while it sometimes makes sense to distinguish between physical and mental aspects of human life, it is neither conceptually nor practically desirable to distinguish between physical and mental health promotion.**

People are physical, thinking beings. Once we have no physical function we are dead. And if we cannot think we might as well be.

The belief that it is appropriate to have health workers specialise exclusively in the physical **or** the mental is a pervasive curse of the Western world. We have created an unreal taxonomy – a system of classifying ourselves that is against our true nature. We have come to think that it is acceptable – praiseworthy indeed – that a surgeon should not concern himself with a patient's anxieties, that scientists should conduct research without pausing to think about the implications for general human well-being, and that a psychiatrist can prescribe medication for presumed chemical imbalances in the brain with hardly a pause for reflection on a patient's life circumstances.

Nursing should not perpetuate this corruption. It should bury the error once and for all by stating first what mental health promotion is, and by repeatedly emphasising that this is as basic as it gets. Even though a health promoter may **at times** focus exclusively on either physical or mental obstacles (if those obstacles are so large that they impede all other normal and desirable potentials) there is no sensible distinction between physical health promotion and mental health promotion. The fact that it is at times prudent to focus solely on, say, excessive grief or a physical addiction is a sign that single problems can sometimes be overwhelming – but it is not a proof that our mental and physical worlds are so different from one another that they require separate health promotion disciplines to cope with them.

Consider how ridiculous it would be for a health promoter to focus exclusively on either the grief or the addiction. Grieving has physical consequences – loss of appetite, loss of motivation (a change in behaviour as well as a change in cognition), perhaps even loss of employment and friends. Physical addiction (if it even makes sense to talk of an addiction as exclusively physical) has mental effects – guilt, feelings of failure, disorientation as a result of the use of an addictive substance, and so on.

To make this crystal clear: it is obviously possible to promote health by focusing exclusively on people's mental lives. We try to do this already: in psychotherapy, in education, in encouraging people to read good books, in programmes meant to improve memory, and in countless other ways. But for a health promoter to ignore everything else she might be doing once a crisis has been dealt with just because she is supposed to be a **mental health** promoter is to focus arbitrarily on just one sort of obstacle: and will certainly promote less health than an intelligent effort to provide a solid set of general foundations.

Indeed, as the short discussion of the **foundations theory** has shown – once substantial theory is put forward it quickly becomes apparent that separating mental health promotion from other types **creates** problems that can be avoided by retaining a holistic form of health promotion. The most devastating of these artefacts is thinking of 'mental health issues' as distant from other human concerns. It is, for example, depressingly common to hear health professionals describe correlations between poverty and mental health problems when they take 'mental health problems' to mean only schizophrenia and the like. But of course poverty **itself** is a mental health problem (how many people are happy, fulfilled, creative and at ease in poverty?).

## CONCLUSION

More than any other branch of nursing, mental health nursing exposes the rift between nursing's nurturing instincts and medicine's/society's insistence that aberrant behaviours are contained.

The two outlooks are incompatible. When official nursing bodies find the strength to recommend that mental health nurses practise according to the nursing values articulated in this book, they will create a powerful catalyst for positive change.

# CHAPTER NINE

# Nursing

## SUMMARY

This chapter:

1. Summarises the **limitations of nursing philosophy**.
2. Offers a philosophically and practically sound **framework for nursing practice**.
3. Explains how to use it.

———————— ◆ ————————

## THE STORY SO FAR

The final two chapters of this book propose a **theory of nursing purpose** and a **Universal Code of Practice for Nurses**. In one way, these are radical suggestions (there is nothing so philosophically comprehensive anywhere else in the nursing literature). Yet in another way they are a natural development of nursing philosophy, and it is not unrealistic to hope that at least some nurses – and perhaps even some theorists – will welcome them.

Before these advances are explained, it may be helpful to recall why nursing philosophy has been unable to put forward such substantial ideas independently.

There are two main reasons for nursing philosophy's logjam:

**1. Nursing philosophy is done for purposes other than the clarification of ideas**
Nurses are naturally interested in examining the theoretical basis of their practice. However, the proliferation of nurse theory is also part of a political campaign:

> 1. The foundation of any profession is the development of a specialized body of knowledge

a. In the past, the nursing profession relied on theories from other disciplines, such as medicine . . .
b. For nursing to define its activities and develop its research, it must have its own body of knowledge . . .
d. Like any profession, nursing must have a theoretical base.[125]

In other words, if nursing is to cut loose from medicine's grip it must become an autonomous profession – so it must have a unique theoretical foundation. Unfortunately, the territorially inspired pursuit of this conceptual base has spawned a deluge of dubious philosophy.

## 2. Too many nurse theorists are trying to force nursing philosophy to do the job only analytic philosophy can do

Nursing's impatience for professional standing has meant that hopeful speculations have been accepted (by some nurses) as established philosophical theory. And there are now so many of these speculations – and so many nurse theorists are idolised for making them – that they have become a formidable barrier to real philosophical progress.

In order to do analytic philosophy proper it is now necessary to criticise an extensive body of literature widely respected in nursing. Understandably, up and coming nurse theorists are reluctant to do this – but do it they must if progress is to be made.

Most nursing philosophy is conceptually impotent. For example, Ruby Wesley thinks nursing has 'four conceptual components':

a. *Person* refers to the recipient of nursing care, including physical, spiritual, psychological and sociocultural components
b. *Environment* refers to all the internal and external conditions, circumstances, and influences affecting the person
c. *Health* refers to the degree of wellness or illness experienced by the person
d. *Nursing* refers to the actions, characteristics, and attributes of the individual providing the nursing care[125]

She says that these four concepts constitute a nursing 'metaparadigm', which is:

the organizing conceptual or philosophical framework of a discipline or profession . . .[125]

According to Wesley every nurse theorist agrees about the importance of the 'nursing metaparadigm'. But how could anyone **not** consider persons, environment, health and nursing of central relevance to nursing?

Consider the 'metaparadigm's' components a little more closely:

*Person* refers to the recipient of nursing care, including physical, spiritual, psychological and sociocultural components[125]

It is hard to deny that a person consists of physical, psychological and spiritual components (and harder still to see why anyone would want to). So why say it? Everyone knows that nurses nurse people and that people are complex beings.

It is similarly unhelpful to state that:

*Health* refers to the degree of wellness or illness experienced by the person[125]

Presumably the idea is that 'wellness' and 'illness' form a continuum along which a person's illness increases as his wellness decreases. But, as several authors have pointed out, this notion is simplistic. It is, for instance, possible to feel well and still be unhealthy, and to feel ill and still be healthy.[123]

Once such elementary difficulties are pointed out it is easy enough to see that writing of this kind is not proper philosophy. However, some nursing philosophy is penned so obscurely that it deceives readers who have not been philosophically trained.

Textbooks of nursing theory offer countless examples. For instance, Pearson et al[126] explain that Rosemary Parse based her *Human Becoming* theory[127] on Rogers' work[128] (see also [129,130]). The authors describe Parse's understanding of 'person' in quasi-mystical terms:

> *The human is coexisting while coconstituting rhythmical patterns with the universe* (coexistence, coconstitution and pattern) . . .
> *The human is a living unity continuously coconstituting patterns of relating* (energy field, pattern and coconstitution).
> *The human is transcending multidimensionally with the possibles* (four-dimensionality, situated freedom and openness).
>
> Parse thus describes the person as an indivisible, responsible being, forever changing and growing as a result of interaction with the universe. Interaction with others and the universe is a rhythmical pattern of closeness and distance . . .[126]
> (The words in brackets are inserted by Pearson et al, to refer to the same or similar ideas in Rogers' work.)

This is seemingly impressive stuff. However, according to Wesley:

> *Four dimensionality* refers to a non-linear domain without spatial or temporal attributes; its boundaries are imaginary and continuously fluctuating[125]

And:

> Integrality refers to the continuous and mutual interaction between the human and environmental fields. Because the two fields are inseparable, both have the same features. As a result, sequential changes in life processes take place at the same time and in the same manner in both fields. These life processes occur as continuous revisions.[125]

As far as it is possible to comprehend any of this, it means that the person disappears. Logic insists that neither Parse nor Rogers can talk about persons because they have dissolved them into a universe without boundaries. If the human and environmental 'fields' are 'inseparable' and 'have the same features' then they are not different – they are identical. Logically, whenever 'you' (if indeed there can be a 'you') nurse a human being you must, according to these nurse philosophers, be nursing the universe too.

## NURSING MODELS AND PROCESSES

There are less high-flown ideas about nursing, usually described as nursing models or processes. But these are mostly descriptions of strategies useful for anyone – doctors, porters, care assistants, neighbours, strangers – who would like to help others deal with health problems. Usually the methods require technical skills, but more often than not they are life skills marshalled by the nurse theorist.

For example, Sister Callista Roy's model of nursing is thoughtful, orderly and practically useful – though certainly not special to nursing.

Here's how Pearson et al describe it:

> The model is largely based on systems theory . . . Roy related adaptation level theory, from the field of psychophysics, to the world of nursing. The view from which the model has been developed is of the individual, as a whole system, responding or *adapting* to changes or *stimuli*. These stimuli are within the individual or in the surrounding environment.[126]

Roy breaks this idea down into components that can be systematically applied by nurses. For example, the 'environment' is said to be an 'internal and external stimulus' which can be divided into three further categories: **focal** (those things which immediately affect a person – an infection or a new baby for instance), **contextual** (other co-present stimuli – anaemia, poor housing or social isolation, perhaps) and **residual** (a person's beliefs, attitudes and traits).[126]

In order to adapt to the environment people 'have certain needs which they endeavour to meet'.[126] These are, **physiological** (the body's structure and function), **self-concept** (how the person thinks of herself), **role**, and **interdependence** (the balance between dependence on others and independence). Pearson explains:

> In Roy's view the purpose of nursing is to help people to adapt to stimuli in any of the four categories identified in order to help them free energy to respond to other stimuli. She suggests that a goal statement should include the behaviour which is to be changed and the direction of the change. She also emphasises that since it is the behaviour of the patient or client which is to be changed, he or she must be involved in identifying goals whenever possible.[126]

Roy's interpretation of nursing lends itself to practical planning (the 'care plan'). For example, on admission a patient can be assessed according to Roy's 'categories of need' (physiological, self-concept and so on), and the impact of the patient's problem on these needs can in turn be assessed according to the categories **focal**, **contextual** and **residual**. So, for instance, if a patient is admitted with a shoulder injury the nurse might make the following record:

---

### Physiological

**Patient behaviour**: Pain and 50% loss of movement in left shoulder

**Focal stimulus**: Difficulty in carrying bags and pain when moving arm

**Contextual stimulus**: No car, has to carry computer and other heavy bags on shoulder for 2 miles daily

**Residual**: Has lived alone for many years and values independence greatly

*continues*

---

┌─ *continued* ──────────

### Role function

**Patient behaviour**: Upset and frustrated by the disability

**Focal stimulus**: Pain and impaired movement

**Contextual**: Unable to swim – swimming is a central component of his life and self-image ...

And so on.

◆

Models such as Roy's are both sensible and practical, partly because they are rooted in nursing experience and do not depend on philosophical fancy. Were nursing to combine these practical insights with decent analytic philosophy the conceptual congestion would dissipate.

## WHAT MORE IS NEEDED?

Nursing desires a unique role. It has been trying to get it through a form of philosophy not equipped to achieve it. Nursing has been trying to find out which **essential quality** makes it special (care? advocacy? ethics? holism?). But there is no more progress to be made this way.

Nursing has been asking the wrong question. In order to understand the nature of nursing one must ask: **'what is nursing's purpose?'**, not **'what is nursing's essence?'**

> ... with practical disciplines such as nursing or ethics, we should not ask first 'what is it?' but rather 'what is it for?'[131]

We need to work out what nurses ought to be doing and how they ought to be doing it. And in order to do this we do indeed need an 'organising framework' – but we need one derived from an understanding of nursing's purpose, built by analytic philosophy.

Such a framework is possible only if philosophical analysis is properly done on all its components (hence the analyses offered in **Chapters Two** to **Eight**), and only if the framework is constructed logically, in a way that makes practical sense.

*SECTION TWO*

## A PHILOSOPHICALLY AND PRACTICALLY SOUND FRAMEWORK FOR NURSING PRACTICE

This section proposes a flexible hierarchy of nursing purposes, made up of nursing's most favoured concepts. These concepts are expressed as **nursing tasks**.

In this hierarchy the higher purposes govern the lower ones. It is impossible to formulate the lower purposes properly (Why these? What is their point? What do they mean? How can they be applied in practice?) unless the higher goals have been systematically and explicitly expressed.

## AN INTRODUCTORY EXAMPLE

First – to help understand why it is so important to have a conceptual hierarchy in nursing – **Figure 14** gives a (debatable) example from another field. At first sight it may seem that these tasks are of equal importance and interchangeable – or that they are a compatible cluster, each necessary to and supporting the others. It may seem as if **Task 3** – for example – is just as important as **Task 2**. It might possibly even appear more significant.

It might seem to some teachers that the primary purpose of their work is to 'encourage a climate in which children feel safe and able to ask questions and challenge assumptions'. However, though this is a worthy aim (in my opinion) **it cannot be the primary teaching goal because it prompts questions which must be answered to gain a satisfactory explanation of the point of teaching**. For example, it prompts the queries: '**Why** is it important to encourage children to ask questions?', '**What** sort of questions should they be encouraged to ask?' and '**Why** is it desirable that children challenge assumptions?'. These questions cannot be answered by **Task 3**, nor can they be answered by **Tasks 4–6**. In order to answer them it is necessary to refer to **Tasks 1** and **2**.

The reason schoolteachers should 'encourage a climate in which children feel safe and able to ask questions and challenge assumptions' is that this is necessary in order to enable children to 'assess information critically' **(Task 2)**, and the reason why **Task 2** is necessary is – of course – **Task 1**: 'to ensure that all children become informed adult participants in the development of the social systems in which they will live'.

In fact the hierarchy is not quite as simple as it seems in **Figure 14**. If children are not reasonably physically and mentally fit **(Task 4)** they cannot inhabit the **Task 3** climate. Furthermore, they will not be able to assimilate information **(Task 5)**, nor will they be able to master the tools with which to analyse it **(Task 6)**. However, even if the children are physically and mentally fit **(Task 4)**, **Tasks 1, 2** and **3** cannot be achieved without the necessary information **(Task 5)** and the analytic tools **(Task 6)**.

Given this, a more accurate hierarchy of schooling purposes might look like **Figure 15**.

**Tasks 4, 5,** and **6** are now divided into **Tasks 3a** and **3b** and **4**. **Task 3a** is roughly equally important to **Task 3b** and **4** feeds them all (but is itself partially dependent upon **3a** and **3b**). This is a loose hierarchy only (and of course many other sources outside school feed each task) but it is nonetheless practically and philosophically helpful.

Note also that it is possible to ask further questions about **Task 1** (**the pinnacle task**) (for instance, 'Why is it important for all children to become informed and participating citizens?' 'Why shouldn't some children merely be good labourers and producers?'). However, in any hierarchy of values there will be at least one unjustified prejudice – at least one point where the person who has set up the hierarchy makes a

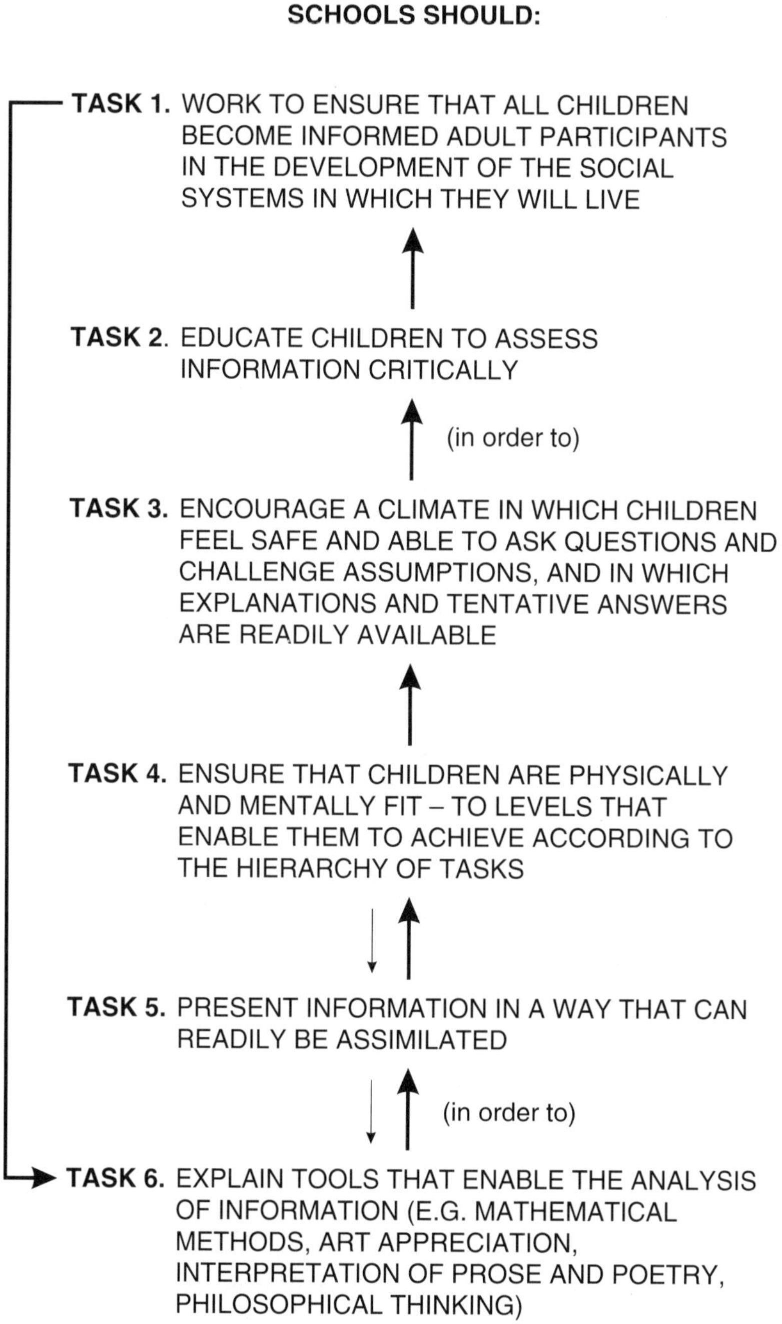

**SCHOOLS SHOULD:**

**TASK 1.** WORK TO ENSURE THAT ALL CHILDREN
BECOME INFORMED ADULT PARTICIPANTS
IN THE DEVELOPMENT OF THE SOCIAL
SYSTEMS IN WHICH THEY WILL LIVE

**TASK 2.** EDUCATE CHILDREN TO ASSESS
INFORMATION CRITICALLY

 (in order to)

**TASK 3.** ENCOURAGE A CLIMATE IN WHICH CHILDREN
FEEL SAFE AND ABLE TO ASK QUESTIONS AND
CHALLENGE ASSUMPTIONS, AND IN WHICH
EXPLANATIONS AND TENTATIVE ANSWERS
ARE READILY AVAILABLE

**TASK 4.** ENSURE THAT CHILDREN ARE PHYSICALLY
AND MENTALLY FIT – TO LEVELS THAT
ENABLE THEM TO ACHIEVE ACCORDING TO
THE HIERARCHY OF TASKS

**TASK 5.** PRESENT INFORMATION IN A WAY THAT CAN
READILY BE ASSIMILATED

 (in order to)

**TASK 6.** EXPLAIN TOOLS THAT ENABLE THE ANALYSIS
OF INFORMATION (E.G. MATHEMATICAL
METHODS, ART APPRECIATION,
INTERPRETATION OF PROSE AND POETRY,
PHILOSOPHICAL THINKING)

**Figure 14** A schooling hierarchy. The arrows indicate a flexible relationship, but a hierarchical one nevertheless. The arrows between 5 and 6 and 4 and 5 are reversible, as shown

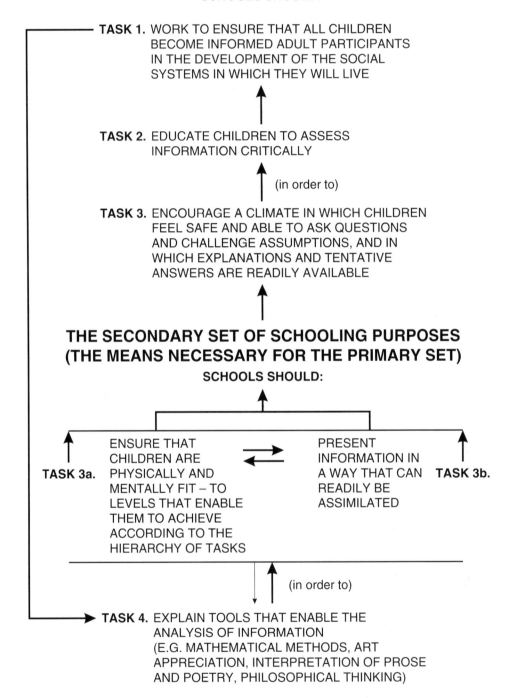

**Figure 15** A schooling hierarchy divided into primary and secondary purposes

stand and says – 'this just is intrinsically good' (this is the **ethical commitment** explained in **Chapter Ten**).

## CONCEPTUAL HIERARCHIES ARE HELPFUL

Hierarchies of purpose can be spelt out in any field of human endeavour. They are instructive because:

1. They enable people to see the point of what they are doing more clearly.
2. They help people organise their practical activities purposefully, logically and efficiently.
3. People – even professional people – do not always work according to the same hierarchy of purposes. Unless the hierarchies are spelled out, we may labour under the misapprehension that we are pulling in the same direction when we are not. Spell out the supposed hierarchies and at least we can see where we disagree.

**Figure 16** is a second illustrative example. This time two different hierarchies of purpose are proposed. In each case, as with the hierarchies of schooling purpose, the lower goals make sense only in relation to the higher ones (within each 'marriage hierarchy'), and the **pinnacle task** directs and cements the rest.

For example, in both cases the partners wish to have a happy marriage above all else (their **Tasks 1** – the **pinnacle tasks**). However, **Partner One**'s personal interests are valuable only in so far as they enable him sufficient freedom and happiness to be totally committed to the well-being of his partner, while **Partner Two**'s interests are valuable first for their own sake.

Each partner could do worse than try to spell out the hierarchies, to see where – if anywhere – there is potential trouble. This way each will be able:

1. To see the point of what they are doing more clearly.
2. To organise their daily activities logically and purposefully, if possible to achieve shared goals.
3. To see where they disagree about the point of their marriage – which is surely better than labouring under the misperception that they are pulling in the same direction when they are not.

## NURSING'S CONCEPTUAL HIERARCHY

The same is true of nursing.

Most nurse philosophers support a hierarchy of sorts, at least in so far as they offer up a particular notion as nursing's driving force – caring, advocacy, morality, the patient, holistic nursing and so on – and then sub-divide it. To offer this alternative hierarchy is not to say that the nurse theorists are wrong. In the realm of values there are no absolutely right and wrong answers – if a nurse says the point of nursing is to care, or

# IN MARRIAGE

## PARTNER ONE'S HIERARCHY

### I SHOULD:

**TASK 1.** BE UNCONDITIONALLY LOVING AND
SUPPORTIVE TO MY PARTNER

**TASK 2.** PLACE MY PERSONAL INTERESTS BELOW
THOSE OF THE PARTNERSHIP, WHERE THE
TWO SETS CONFLICT

**TASK 3.** PURSUE PERSONAL PROJECTS AND
PERSONAL HAPPINESS

**TASK 4.** WORK TO KEEP PHYSICALLY AND MENTALLY
FIT

## PARTNER TWO'S HIERARCHY

### I SHOULD:

**TASK 1.** PLACE MY PERSONAL INTERESTS FIRST,
SO LONG AS THEY ARE NOT
DETRIMENTAL TO THE MARRIAGE

**TASK 2.** BE LOVING AND SUPPORTIVE TO MY PARTNER

**TASK 3.** PURSUE PERSONAL PROJECTS AND
PERSONAL HAPPINESS

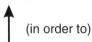

(in order to)

**TASK 4.** WORK TO KEEP PHYSICALLY AND MENTALLY FIT

**Figure 16**    Two marriage hierarchies

to advocate, then she is right because this is what she believes to be of utmost importance and this (presumably) is how she organises her own nursing care.

However, I am arguing the following:

1. **That some of the purposes offered by some nursing theorists are inadequate because they require further justification** – either conceptually (why care like this?) or practically (how does one consistently achieve patient dignity?).
2. **That a hierarchy of nursing purpose with work for health at its head – as the pinnacle nursing task – makes philosophical, logical, political and practical sense** – in the end there are only two questions for nurses to answer: 'What is health?' and 'How can I create it?' Because of their interest in philosophy and their determination to care humanely, nurses are the best placed of all health workers to ask these questions seriously, to develop a considered view on them, and to try to put them consistently into practice. As they answer them, the other nursing values fall into place – and can be interpreted and applied intelligently without the many gaps in explanation which presently require an act of faith to accept.
3. **That the hierarchy of nursing purpose proposed in Figure 17 can create a practically meaningful nursing Code of Practice.**
4. **That this hierarchy can be clearly explained to nursing students, without resort to mystifying philosophical notions, appeal to intuition, or recourse to rhetoric or emotional pleading.**
5. **That therefore the hierarchy can be accepted or rejected on explicit, clearly argued grounds.**
6. **That the hierarchy, its moral importance, and what it means in practice can be readily explained to patients, who will then know where their nurses stand.**

Notice that there is no place for ethics in this hierarchical scheme. This is because the whole of nursing practice is a moral endeavour: **nursing is an ethical enterprise.**[15]

And that – in sum – is all there is. Of course there is much more – a world more – to practising as a nurse according to this conceptual hierarchy, but this is nevertheless a beautifully condensed way for nurses to remind themselves of their basic priorities (if they share this understanding of nursing purpose, of course).

Like the schooling hierarchy, there are two sets of nursing purposes – a **primary** one and a **secondary** one. The **primary** set is governed directly by the notion of health (the **pinnacle task** of the entire hierarchy) which should guide nurses as they work out which sort of care to offer, and help them carefully and specifically to plot how to promote patient dignity.

Without the **primary** set, the **secondary** set is open to wide interpretation at best, and at worst is meaningless.

Note that these are **comprehensively meaningful** notions, not vague aspirations. **Task 1** – work for health – does not mean something amorphous like 'work for complete, physical, social and mental well-being'. Instead, it is a well-argued and well-specified explanation of how one might go about influencing the factors that make up other people's health (see **Chapter Eight** and *Health Promotion*[7] for example).

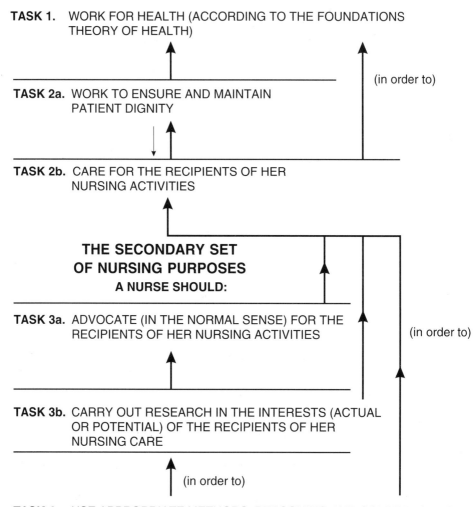

**IN NURSING**

**THE PRIMARY SET OF
NURSING PURPOSES**

**A NURSE SHOULD:**

**TASK 1.**   WORK FOR HEALTH (ACCORDING TO THE FOUNDATIONS
THEORY OF HEALTH)

(in order to)

**TASK 2a.**   WORK TO ENSURE AND MAINTAIN
PATIENT DIGNITY

**TASK 2b.**   CARE FOR THE RECIPIENTS OF HER
NURSING ACTIVITIES

**THE SECONDARY SET
OF NURSING PURPOSES**
**A NURSE SHOULD:**

**TASK 3a.**   ADVOCATE (IN THE NORMAL SENSE) FOR THE
RECIPIENTS OF HER NURSING ACTIVITIES

(in order to)

**TASK 3b.**   CARRY OUT RESEARCH IN THE INTERESTS (ACTUAL
OR POTENTIAL) OF THE RECIPIENTS OF HER
NURSING CARE

(in order to)

**TASK 4.**   USE APPROPRIATE METHODS, REASONING AND COMMUNICATION

**Figure 17**   Nursing's conceptual hierarchy. The arrow – in either direction – means 'in order to'

**Task 1** is a hierarchy in itself (see **Figure 13** in **Chapter Eight**). By doing it a nurse can
decide which practical nursing sub-tasks are required and in what order to do them –
so seeking an efficient cure for a patient's problem, for example. However, she can
also do more. She can consider the other conditions which make up people's health –
their basic needs, their environment, their emotions, their comprehension, their
spirituality – and do what she can about these too.

The **pinnacle task** works to organise and give character to the lower goals because it offers essential guidance about what sort of caring is required and what is needed to maintain dignity in a particular situation, for instance.

Here is an illustrative example:

## HOW NURSING'S CONCEPTUAL HIERARCHY WORKS

Consider how **nursing's conceptual hierarchy** can help nurses:

a. organise nursing tasks
b. recognise that advocacy in the **normal sense** (for example) is not the **pinnacle task**, but part of the secondary set of nursing purposes
c. determine how to act in difficult situations.

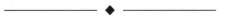

---

### CASE EIGHT

### Charles' Stroke

Charles is 80 and has had a right-hemisphere haemorrhagic infarct. He has completely lost the use of his left leg. His right arm and leg are still sound but his left arm and side are very weak. He can speak, but only with great difficulty. It is not easy to understand him.

Charles is a retired boiler-maker, well known for being a cheerful, harmless soul. He has two adult sons who both live a couple of car-hours away.

Before his stroke he was living routinely in a council house, with his wife, two years his junior. She (Mary) has always been in charge of the major household decisions. Charles would have liked to have had more of a say, but Mary is a born leader and smarter than him, so Charles gave this ambition up a long time ago. Charles' passion was gardening – he grew prize tomatoes and chrysanthemums – a hobby which kept him happily occupied for much of the day.

Two weeks ago Mary woke to find Charles immobile by her side in their bed, tears running from his eyes. She guessed what had happened straightaway, called the doctor and an hour later Charles was in an ambulance on the way to hospital.

Kate is one of Charles' nurses, and a devoted nurse advocate. At first she wasn't sure whether he would survive, but she can see he is recovering slowly – at least physically. Kate's just heard that Charles' physiotherapy is to be increased, with a view to significant rehabilitation – even to getting him walking again. As she chirpily tells Charles this

*continues*

┌─ *continued* ─────────────────────────────────

latest news he fixes her with a brutal glare – 'SSfuck sssthat,' he dribbles. Kate is shocked, but Charles forces on. 'I'm sno ussse na. No phhss … no mrre phssthhry. Fththuuc off.' Then he shuts his eyes.

───────────  ◆  ───────────

Charles' reaction places Kate in a difficult position. She is an experienced nurse and she thinks it possible that in time Charles may recover enough to be able to walk around the house (and his garden) using a frame. Perhaps he might do even better than this, if he has a will to.

Kate has become rather fond of Charles and his devoted wife and would like to help him – both of them – rehabilitate. Kate wants to encourage Charles to undergo the physiotherapy, yet she also wants to advocate for him, which for her means to:

**speak on behalf of Charles as Charles perceives his interests** (see **Chapter Two**)

What is she to do?

## WHY ADVOCACY CANNOT BE THE PINNACLE TASK

To advocate in the **normal sense**:

  i. clashes with Kate's intuition
 ii. offers neither Kate nor Charles the opportunity to reflect on what is best
iii. fails to do justice to the complexity of the situation
 iv. offers no opportunity for ethical analysis
  v. (in this case at least) may lead to significant and avoidable harm.

Advocacy is part of the secondary set because it does not – in itself – offer a justification for advocacy. Once the primary set of nursing concepts is in place it is clear that the question 'should I advocate?' can be answered intelligently and sensitively only by considering it as subsidiary to the intent to care and nurture, the wish to ensure patient dignity and the desire to bring about the greatest possible health for all concerned.

This is obvious on examining any practical case. In Kate's situation, she has various **choices**, which she might lay out like this:

1. I will seek to achieve whatever Charles wants (**blind advocacy**).
2. I will seek to achieve what is in Charles' best interest (**Kate's intuition**).
3. I will seek to enable Charles to achieve what he decides is in his best interest after he has been provided with the opportunity to think about it more deeply (**foundational health-based advocacy**).

4. Even if Charles still declines physiotherapy after he has had time to think about it I will seek to achieve what I know to be in Charles' best interest (**autonomy creation/ misplaced parentalism**).

In order to seek a **primary justification** she might next address three questions – one from each of the three primary levels:

**Task 2b: How should I care for Charles?**
**Task 2a: How can I ensure Charles' dignity?**
**Task 1: How can I best work for Charles' health?**

**Task 2b. How Should I Care for Charles?**

Recall the **four types of care**:

---

**The View That Caring Implies Emotional Involvement**

If a person is to care properly for another, she should be 'emotionally involved with' him.

**Caring as Performing Conventional Activities of Care**

This form involves carrying out activities which conventionally constitute 'caring for a sick person'. In this way it is possible for the nurse to care automatically, without having any feeling of involvement with the person being cared for.

**Caring as Being Prudent**

This form involves caring by exhibiting those actions most likely to be productive (taking care to do a good job, in other words). This does not require a direct personal interest in another person.

**Portraying Caring**

Caring by deliberately portraying a personal interest in someone, in order to bring about a desired result, even though the carer does not actually feel an attachment.

---

The question now is: which of these forms should Kate invoke? Though it goes without saying in this case that Kate should **prudently perform** her **conventional duties**, it is not clear whether she should become (or continue to be) **emotionally involved** with Charles, nor whether she should **portray care** (if she is not involved, or if she loses emotional involvement).

If one reflects on the substance of either policy – on what it might mean for Kate and Charles – it becomes obvious that caring alone is not enough. However much Kate cares she is no closer to a solution to her problem, namely: should she do what Charles asks or should she try to encourage Charles along a path she believes to be best for him? If she decides to **portray care**, the question remains: To what end should I portray care? And if she does become emotionally attached to Charles this does not mean she will automatically do what he asks, indeed it might make the opposite more likely. If she bonds to him it could be more painful for her to see him relinquishing the chance to live a worthwhile life once more, and so she might try harder to bring him round to her way of thinking.

**Task 2a. How Can I Ensure Charles' dignity?**

Thinking about dignity can help Kate choose which caring approach to adopt. Remember that we may lack dignity:

> **In circumstances ill-fitted to our competencies (Type 1)**

and

> **In circumstances in which we are normally capable, but where we fail to achieve what we routinely would (Type 2)** (see **Chapter Four**)

Charles presently lacks dignity on both counts. He has never experienced these circumstances before and is barely competent to deal with them. Furthermore, he is failing to achieve what he normally would even in those few circumstances where he is normally capable (deciding what he wants, asking for it, and having his wishes met, for example).

This helps Kate because she now has clear choices. She can try to improve Charles' **circumstances**, or his **competencies**, or **both**. This is a practically meaningful choice because Charles is surely in one of these categories:

**1iii. He is in circumstances ill-fitted to his competencies, and is suffering a serious loss of dignity.**

Or

**1iv. He is in circumstances ill-fitted to his competencies and is suffering a devastating loss of dignity.**

Kate should now ask: '**Can I change Charles' circumstances?**' and '**Can I change Charles' competencies?**' for these are the only ways in which his dignity can be restored.

Now Kate has something substantial to work on. Charles' **wall of dignity** (see **Figure 6** in **Chapter Four**) has collapsed and needs rebuilding. Kate must make efforts to repair it.

**Task 1: How Can I Best Work for Charles' Health?**
Work to improve Charles' dignity is also work for his health (**work for health** is the **pinnacle task** of **Nursing's Conceptual Hierarchy**). So how best to work to improve Charles' dignity depends upon Kate's deliberation about what is most lacking in Charles' health, and what she is most able to provide. Without the support of a theory of health, working for Charles' dignity could be a rather empty task. Furthermore, it could stall at precisely the same conundrum – do I do what **I** think is best for Charles' dignity or do I do what **he** thinks is best for his dignity. Only by thinking at the stage higher – at the level of work for health in the hierarchy – can this problem be resolved.

As Kate asks: '**Can I change Charles' circumstances?**' '**Can I change Charles' competencies?**' she is asking, '**Which foundations can I work on?**' In other words,

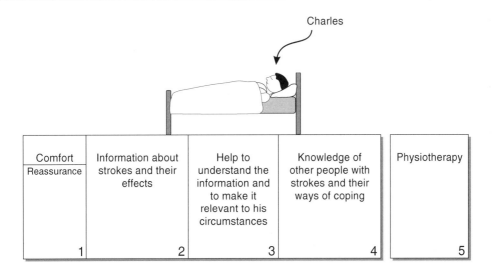

**Figure 18** Charles' foundations through Kates' eyes. Note that this image indicates the foundations to be worked on or created, not as they are at present

Kate has to decide – as the 'airport departure board' (see **Chapter Eight**) clicks over for Charles – do I focus on:

Charles' basic needs (Box One)?
The information available to him (Box Two)?
His education – his means of assimilating information (Box Three)?
His sense of belonging (and sense of self) (Box Four)?

And/or

His special needs of the moment (Box Five)?

If Kate were to decide to concentrate only on Box 5 she would be inclined to press ahead with the physiotherapy whatever Charles says – but this would be to miss almost everything that is humane in working for health.

**Figure 18** shows one simple way in which Kate might view Charles' foundations.

Note that the backcloth for Kate's analysis is ethical reflection. So she also uses the **Caring Grid**:

Because she is able to use these tools Kate quickly sees that the basic tension is between:

**I should nurture this person/these people (1)** (create autonomy).
**I should take this person's/these people's views as seriously as I take my own (2)** (respect autonomy).

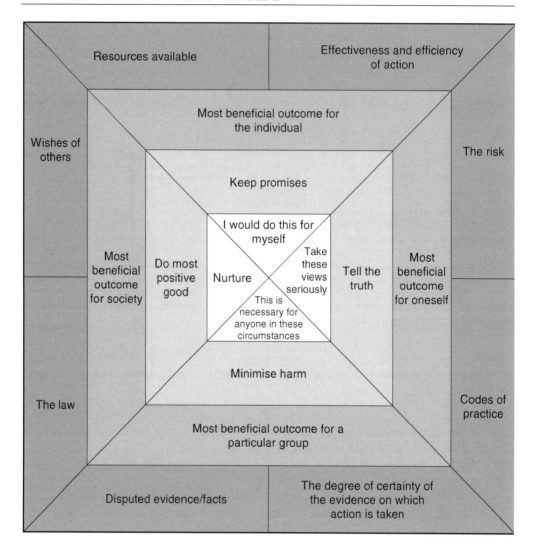

## WHAT DOES KATE DECIDE?

Kate fills out Charles' foundations image as in **Figure 18**, deciding that the best way to care for him is to be completely honest about everything, including her feelings for him and his wife and her frustration that he will not do what she knows to be best for him. She shows the image to Charles and explains it to him (note that the sizes of the boxes are not uniform – some are bigger than others, reflecting their relative importance, in Kate's view). She asks if she can also show it to Mary, so that they can check out whether their perception of the situation is the same as Kate's. Charles agrees and they all work on it.

It transpires in discussion that Kate's foundations image is very different from Charles', and that Mary's is different again. Their images are shown in **Figures 19** and **20**.

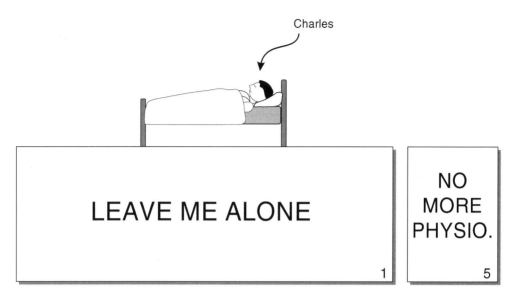

**Figure 19** Charles' foundations through Charles' eyes. Note that this image reflects the foundations as Charles sees them at the moment

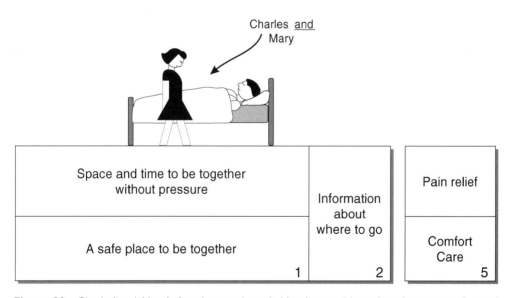

**Figure 20** Charles' and Mary's foundations through Mary's eyes. Note that this image reflects the foundations to be worked on or created, not as they are at present

Kate has emphasised boxes 2, 3, 4 and 5 – particularly 2 and 4 since she believes Charles needs most to understand how he might improve. Charles has emphasised Box 1 alone – he does not need anything else. However much he gets better he will not be able to be the person he was before. He cannot pursue Charles' life goals any more, so his life has lost its meaning. He would prefer to be left alone with his memories and when nature takes its course he will accept that.

Unlike Charles, Mary sees the focus of concern as the pair of them, a married couple. Because of this it is not for her to express an individual view – however much she would like to cry out that Charles must do what the nurse says – but to express a shared view. She wants Charles back as he was but she knows she cannot ever have him back like this. She also knows – because her boxes 2 and 3 are solid in this respect (her own mother nursed her father in similar circumstances, for several years) – that the impact on her, Charles and their relationship will be immense if he does have the physiotherapy and eventually comes home to be looked after by her. She says – courageously and with enormous sadness – that she agrees with Charles. It is better for them if Charles does not have the physiotherapy – that way they can be together in this short trouble and then Charles will be gone.

Kate is then left with this choice:

iii. I will seek to enable Charles to achieve what he decides is in his best interest after he has been provided with the opportunity to think about it more deeply (**foundations health-based advocacy**).

Or

iv. Even if Charles still declines physiotherapy after he has had time to think about it I will seek to achieve what I know to be in Charles' best interest (**autonomy creation/ misplaced parentalism**).

Kate decides that if she pressed on with her intuition – having done considerable work for health already – she would be crossing the line under (iv) – from **autonomy creation** to **misplaced parentalism** – so she decides to opt for (iii) instead – **health-based advocacy**.

But she needs more practical detail in order to proceed. So she takes her lead from her understanding of dignity.

She sees that:

> **Charles is in circumstances ill-fitted to his competencies and is suffering a devastating loss of dignity.**

She now knows that Charles will not accept the help of a physiotherapist to change his physical (and perhaps mental) circumstances, so she needs to work for health **realistically**. That is, she needs to identify which other circumstances she can now change and which existing competencies she can support and which – if any – new competencies she can provide for Charles and Mary (she has now accepted Mary's view that she is to **work for the health of the couple**).

Consequently, she works with Charles and Mary to find a home outside the hospital for Charles, as near as possible to Mary's house. She also asks them to consider their financial arrangements, and to reflect on spiritual matters. Unfortunately, Charles' consultant does not approve and thinks that he ought to be persuaded to undergo further physiotherapy – so in the end Kate advocates (in the **normal sense**) for Charles and Mary, even though this means she has to advocate a counter-intuitive position.

Eventually the consultant concedes defeat, Charles is placed in a nearby Hospice, and he seems to relax slowly into death. Two weeks later he dies.

Kate is very sad at this. But she is proud of the depth of her thinking. She has applied a thoughtful philosophy of health rather than a vague and fashionable notion that advocacy is central. Even though in one sense the result is the same as if she had simply advocated for Charles straightaway, there is a world of difference. Everything was explicitly stated and reasoned, Kate was able to understand why it was right for her to act against her instinct. Mary and Charles were fully involved in this most important of decisions, and Kate was able to mount a strong, reasoned argument against the consultant's own intuition.

# CHAPTER TEN

# The Universal Ethical Code

## SUMMARY

This chapter:

1. Describes the **Ethics Myth**.
2. Explains that **ethics is everywhere**.
3. Presents a **Universal Ethical Code** for health care.
4. Explains how to use it.
5. Unites the book's themes and analyses.

Note: Since nursing practice takes place entirely within the ethical realm (as explained below) the Code might equally be called THE UNIVERSAL CODE OF PRACTICE or THE UNIVERSAL CODE OF ETHICS. For simplicity it is called THE UNIVERSAL CODE in the remainder of this chapter.

———————— ◆ ————————

*SECTION ONE*

## ETHICS IS EVERYWHERE

## INTRODUCTION

Before concluding that a code of ethics is not useful and should be abandoned, it is important to assess whether expectations for what a code of ethics can and cannot do are reasonable... The challenge is to make a code of ethics into a living document that helps nurses join in the dialogue and discernment about essential ethical issues.[132]

Are we on the wrong track, in terms of our expectations of a code of practice, professional ethics teaching or the wider field of moral philosophy; in our search for clear answers to the ethical problems that arise in clinical practice...?... [W]e are likely to be misguided in assuming that there are always clear, straightforward answers to the ethical problems of clinical practice. However, more than a fleeting acquaintance with the field of ethics may help us to begin to think with greater clarity about what we do and why we do it. The hope is that this may lead to considered, humane practice by design, with the critical understanding and support of our professional peers and employers.[133]

Traditional Codes of Practice command their subjects to abide by their legislation:

> Nurses *shall* ...[134]
>
> All medical practitioners ... *will accept* the following Principles of Ethical Behaviour[135]
>
> A doctor *must practice* his profession uninfluenced by motives of profit[2]
>
> A nurse *is obliged* to treat clients with respect for their individual needs and values[4]
>
> (My italics, in each case.)

Where these moral laws come from, and why practitioners should obey them, is always a mystery.[136]

## A PROFOUND MISPERCEPTION

**Figure 21** shows how most people understand ethics in health care. Ethics and health care practice are thought of as separate domains that only occasionally overlap. Routine clinical practice is considered ethically trouble-free. It just happens – with no need for ethical reflection.

But this is a myth, according to which the social world looks like **Figure 22**. As the myth has it, we live on an iceberg adrift on an unseen ocean. Most of the time most of us see only its tip. This is where we go to work, shop, play, travel, watch television and so on. Occasionally dramatic ethical issues spill out of a hidden crevasse. We see a documentary about fiddled waiting lists, or we hear of resource allocation injustices, or we learn that surgeons have lied to patients.

According to the **Ethics Myth** these ethical crises can be dealt with by applying ethical principles and Codes – do no harm, respect people's choices, act justly and so on. Then – once the problem is safely back in the crevasse – we can get on with the daily routine without giving ethics any further thought.

Of course we know there are deeper things to ponder – political matters, religious questions, the impact of science on our lives. And we are also aware of our basic drives to survive, to protect those we love and to succeed in life.

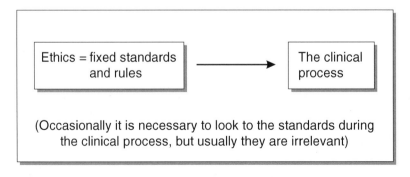

**Figure 21**   A false understanding of ethics in health care

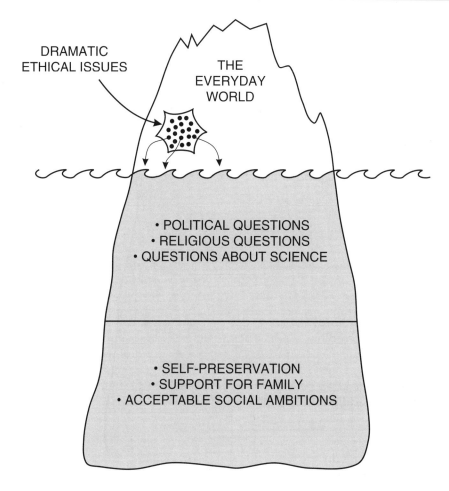

**Figure 22** The moral world according to the Ethics Myth

But on the **Ethics Myth** these lower levels are not of ethical concern. Ethical issues occur only where they can be seen – everything else is given.

## A CONVENIENT FICTION

The **Ethics Myth** is a convenient fiction for those who like things the way they are.

There is a better way to understand ethics. It is not **the** right way (such a proposition about any set of ethical principles is impossible to justify). But it is both more humane and more plausible than the **Myth**.

**Figure 23** gives a clearer view of the iceberg. Though the top looks roughly the same, the lower segments are different. On this interpretation **the entire social world is the ethical realm** – the whole iceberg has ethical content. Seen like this ethics is not a

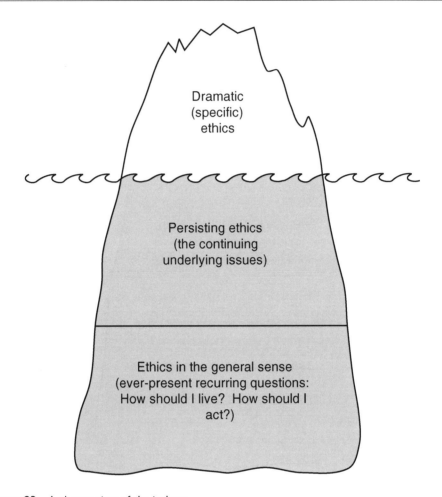

**Figure 23**   A clearer view of the iceberg

special subject at the iceberg's tip, rather **ethics is like blood**. It is part of everything we do.

For example, beneath the dramas about who should get a scarce therapy, there are **persisting issues** about the funding of health systems and the role of private capital in the pricing and availability of life-saving commodities.

Furthermore, what we each choose to do about rationing is an ever-present ethical concern. Say I'm a nurse, should I discriminate between patients or should I refuse to co-operate with an unfair system? Should I explain my beliefs to patients refused dialysis? Should I tell them what I think is fair? Should I campaign for what I believe in or should I hold onto my job even if it means I behave in a way I think is wrong?

If I am a patient should I try to secure an advantage over other patients? Or should I turn down an offer of help on altruistic grounds?

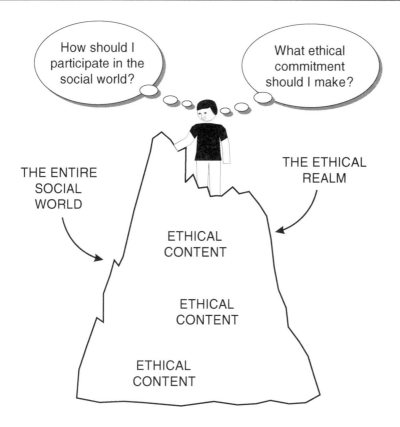

**Figure 24** Ethics is everywhere

It's not just in health care that ethics is everywhere. Ethics is a pervasive phenomenon of human life – **every human action that can affect one or more of us has ethical content**.

Because we live with others in an ethical realm we constantly encounter ethical situations, whether or not we perceive them as such. Whether we realise it or not, being pleasant, unpleasant (or anything else) to people during a Saturday morning trip around the local supermarket are actions with **ethical content** because they have the potential to produce different consequences. If I go out of my way to be friendly I may improve someone else's experience, if only a little. If I scurry about concentrating on the shelves, deliberately distancing myself from other people then I miss a chance to make life's experience better, and I may contribute to someone else's alienation.

In health care – probably more than any other work – it is easier to see that even something habitually dismissed as trivial – a smile for instance – is within the **ethical realm**. A condescending or off-hand smile offered to a sensitive and vulnerable patient may be damaging, while a sincere smile of welcome will probably help put a patient at her ease.

When you see the iceberg like this, the world looks different. On the **Ethics Myth** everything is taken for granted – since we can make little or no ethical difference why should we even try? But if **ethics is everywhere** then everything we do must make an ethical difference.

If what you do in the supermarket – or anywhere else – bothers you then you are on the way to making an **ethical commitment**. Since the founding question of ethics is **how should I conduct my life in the presence of other lives?** your ethical challenge – at any time and in any place – is to work out what **commitment to living** to make.

## CONVENTIONAL CODES HAVE GOT IT WRONG

Conventional Codes of Ethics have done a devastating disservice to how people understand ethics. The problem is not the duties these Codes put forward (as we have seen, they are always vague and general, and easy enough to agree with *prima facie*). Rather it is because they are put forward as rules – commandments that their ethically unaware subjects must obey.

As a result, Codes of Ethics ossify thought by trapping it inside grand declarations. The worst Codes are the antithesis of ethical analysis.

However, the **Universal Code** is unique. At first sight its **six items** look routine – but it understands **morality** and **work for health** differently from other Codes, and comprehensively supports nurses (and others) in their **practical reasoning**.

The **Universal Code** fosters intelligent reflection. It never tells practitioners what to do.

*SECTION TWO*

# THE UNIVERSAL CODE

# WHAT IS A CODE?

Like the other words discussed in this book, 'code' has more than one sense. It is commonly used to mean both 'a system of symbols with hidden meaning' (as in a cipher) and 'a set of rules'. These meanings are used simultaneously in the expression 'genetic code', for example, to indicate that there is a code to be discovered and that its rules govern our development.

The **Universal Code** is not a strict set of rules. Rather it is a group of ideas with a limited meaning, which can be arranged by the Code's user as one might arrange a musical score, or as one arranges flowers. The basic materials are always given, but what one does with them is up to the arranger. Choosing to use them imposes a limit on the user, but within this limit she is free (and encouraged) to use her judgement. Not only this, but the user is at liberty to **commit** to the **Universal Code** or not.

The Universal Ethical Code is presented in the following pages.

## THE UNIVERSAL CODE
### (expressed for nursing)

The Universal Code has only **six items**. These are:

1. A NURSE SHOULD WORK FOR HEALTH
2. A NURSE SHOULD WORK TO ENSURE AND MAINTAIN PATIENT DIGNITY
3. A NURSE SHOULD CARE FOR HER PATIENTS
4. A NURSE SHOULD ADVOCATE FOR HER PATIENTS
5. A NURSE SHOULD CARRY OUT RESEARCH IN THE INTERESTS OF THE ACTUAL OR POTENTIAL RECIPIENTS OF HER NURSING
6. A NURSE SHOULD USE APPROPRIATE METHODS, REASONING AND COMMUNICATION

(Note that 'doctor', 'manager', 'care assistant' etc. could be substituted for 'nurse' in this code, since it is possible to express the **Universal Code** for all health workers.)

Cast like this the **Universal Code** looks like any other Code – indeed, it looks like one of the vaguest. However, to use it properly a nurse must:

> a. Understand its source.
> b. Understand what the 6 points imply.
> c. Possess skills sufficient to act on each duty effectively.
> d. Have a working environment that allows her to act on each duty. effectively.
>
> And – of overwhelming importance – a nurse:
>
> e. Must freely choose to commit to the **Universal Code**.

## EXPLANATION

**IF** a nurse understands the nature of nursing as in the following figure, and **IF** she decides she wants to practise according to this understanding, then she will find the **Universal Code** useful in her work.

## I. A NURSE SHOULD WORK FOR HEALTH

The **primary purpose of nursing** is to work for health:

*continues*

*continued*

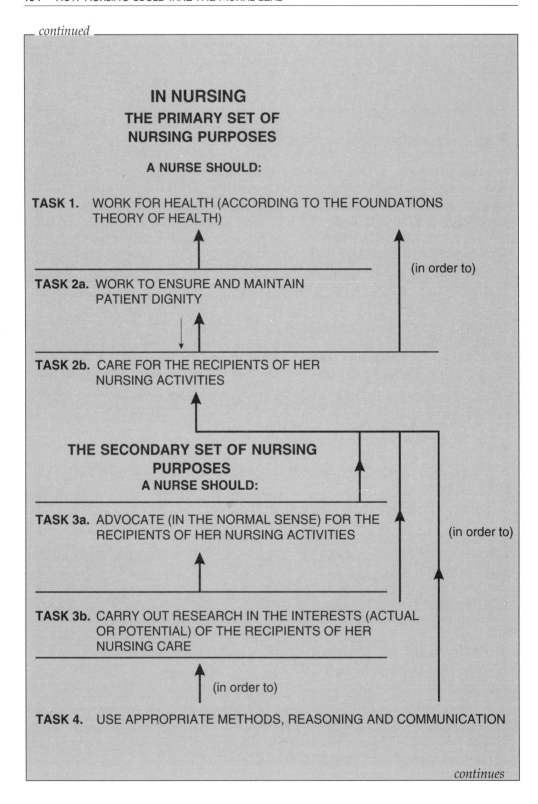

**IN NURSING**
**THE PRIMARY SET OF**
**NURSING PURPOSES**

**A NURSE SHOULD:**

**TASK 1.**   WORK FOR HEALTH (ACCORDING TO THE FOUNDATIONS
THEORY OF HEALTH)

(in order to)

**TASK 2a.**   WORK TO ENSURE AND MAINTAIN
PATIENT DIGNITY

**TASK 2b.**   CARE FOR THE RECIPIENTS OF HER
NURSING ACTIVITIES

**THE SECONDARY SET OF NURSING**
**PURPOSES**
**A NURSE SHOULD:**

**TASK 3a.**   ADVOCATE (IN THE NORMAL SENSE) FOR THE
RECIPIENTS OF HER NURSING ACTIVITIES

(in order to)

**TASK 3b.**   CARRY OUT RESEARCH IN THE INTERESTS (ACTUAL
OR POTENTIAL) OF THE RECIPIENTS OF HER
NURSING CARE

(in order to)

**TASK 4.**   USE APPROPRIATE METHODS, REASONING AND COMMUNICATION

*continues*

*continued*

## Definition

A person's (or group's) (optimum) state of health is equivalent to the state of the conditions which fulfil or enable a person to work to fulfil his or her realistic chosen and biological potentials. Some of these conditions are of the highest importance for all people. Others are variable dependent upon individual abilities and circumstances.

## FRAMEWORK FOR PRACTICE

Health should be thought of like this:

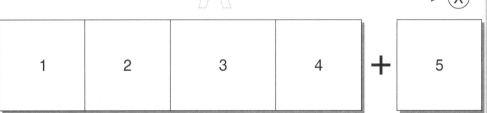

The extent to which a person can function successfully (i.e. the extent to which a person is autonomous) is roughly the extent of his or her health

A person is enabled by the foundations to achieve chosen and biological potentials: if the foundations are complete - in context for the person - then he or she might be said to have optimum health

If the person begins to move towards, arrives at, or is driven towards $(X)$, then additional provision or maintenance of the stage might be necessary

**Figure 12**   An abstract depiction of health

## PRACTICAL WAYS OF WORKING FOR HEALTH

The nurse who wishes to work for health must:

1. Identify a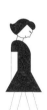
2. Assess the strength of **î**'s foundations for achievement
3. Decide which, if any, require strengthening
4. Identify those she is most competent and able to strengthen
5. Decide – wherever possible in discussion with **î** – which foundations need strengthening first
6. Consider the implications for other people's foundations
7. Act according to her conclusions

*continues*

_continued_

## 2. A NURSE SHOULD WORK TO ENSURE AND MAINTAIN PATIENT DIGNITY

A **primary purpose of nursing** – consequent on working for health – is to promote dignity. This purpose is similar to working for health, though less comprehensive. It prompts the nurse to pay specific attention to a person's **immediate** capabilities and circumstances.

## Definition

Generally speaking:

> A person* will have dignity if he is in a situation where his capabilities can be effectively applied.

Dignity may be defined more specifically like this:

> This person's capabilities are A, B, C…X, Y, Z. She will have dignity in situations where she can exercise these capabilities effectively.
>
> If a nurse wants to promote a person's dignity she must either expand that person's capabilities or improve her circumstances.

Promoting dignity is not the same as promoting health. Dignity must be subjectively experienced whereas health is a set of conditions which need not be known by the person or persons whose health is in question. For example, a new-born baby will have some degree of health but will feel neither dignified nor undignified (see **Chapter Four**).

## FRAMEWORK FOR PRACTICE

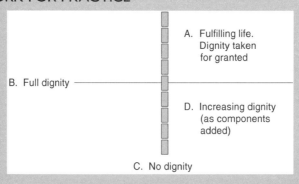

A. Fulfilling life. Dignity taken for granted

B. Full dignity

D. Increasing dignity (as components added)

C. No dignity

---

*A nurse might also work to promote the dignity of a group of people, as is the case with work for health. However – to foster dignity – it usually makes more sense to focus on individuals since dignity is something that has to be felt, and members of a group are unlikely to have identical feelings.

_continues_

*continued*

## PRACTICAL WAYS OF WORKING FOR DIGNITY

A nurse who wishes to promote dignity should:

1. Assess (where possible in consultation with her patient) her patient's position on the graph.
2. If her patient is below **line B** (i.e. if she lacks dignity) she should take an inventory of her patient's past and present capabilities.
3. If her patient is below **line B**, she should take an inventory of her patient's present circumstances.
4. The nurse should then work either to expand that person's capabilities or improve his circumstances, so promoting his dignity.

This may be easier said than done, and sometimes be impossible. But by seeing dignity in this practical way a nurse may be able to make simple yet crucial interventions. For example, if a patient is not presently **capable** of feeding himself he may lack dignity. If so, the nurse who wishes to promote dignity should (if possible) either teach him a technique or provide a tool that will enable him to eat independently again. Failing that, she must find out from the patient precisely which **circumstances** are causing his lack of dignity (a very public situation? Food that is difficult to eat?) and try to improve them.

Or it might be that a nurse notices that a patient is always despondent before visiting time. If so she might ask why (to check out if a mismatch between **capability** and **circumstance** is adversely affecting patient dignity). If she finds out that the patient feels powerless to control who she sees and who she doesn't (a capacity she has previously enjoyed without question) she could – in order to promote dignity – devise a scheme that allows the patient to arrange visits by invitation.

## 3. A NURSE SHOULD CARE FOR HER PATIENTS

A further **primary nursing purpose** is to care for patients.

## Definition

> **In order to care a person must have a concern for something or somebody (she must have an object of care and some interest in it).**

## FRAMEWORK FOR PRACTICE

It is possible to care in different ways as we saw in **Figure 3**.

The first task for the nurse who wishes to care for her patients is to decide **which sort of caring is most appropriate**. In order to do this she will have to ask: **how**

*continues*

*continued*

**can I most effectively work for health?** so making reference to the **pinnacle nursing task.**

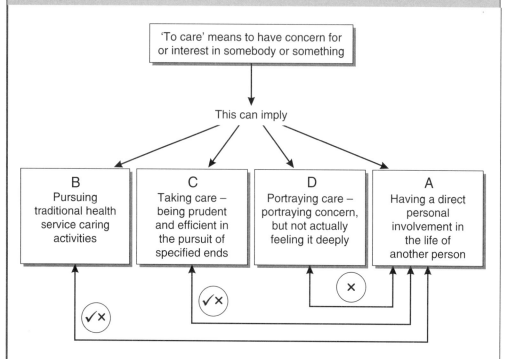

The carer constantly faces a fundamental question, namely:
Why should I choose A, B, C or D – or some combination?

However much she cares she is unable to decide unless she has a
governing theory – a theory beyond 'the ethics of care' – to help her do so

## PRACTICAL WAYS OF CARING FOR PATIENTS

The **Universal Code** is not meant to impede spontaneous caring. Since nurses are not robots they do not always need to check out which sort of care to deliver to patients. Very often their instincts lead them naturally to create health.

However, there are sometimes situations in which it is unclear whether one sort of caring or another is advisable. In such circumstances it is important that the nurse thinks analytically in order to ascertain which form of caring will most promote health.

Caring is a central component of nursing practice. However, a nurse's caring sometimes needs to be guided by an explicit understanding of the reasons why she ought to care.

*continues*

*continued*

If she subscribes to the **Universal Code** she can ensure her care is always directed efficiently toward the achievement of health, and is at least potentially dignifying. For example, even though she finds a patient's racist views offensive a nurse who subscribes to **foundational nursing** will want to work to create more health for him. This will mean both treating his illness (by **taking care** and **pursuing traditional health service activities**) and also providing more general foundations – including information to correct any false beliefs about race he might have, if the nurse considers this a health priority. It will also mean **pretending to be concerned about him**, even though she does not feel concern for him, if doing so will reinforce his foundations.

## 4. A NURSE SHOULD ADVOCATE FOR HER PATIENTS

**A secondary nursing purpose** is to advocate for patients (in the normal sense of advocacy).

## Definition

> **An advocate speaks on behalf of some other person (or persons), as that person perceives his interests.**

**An advocate supports people by taking their side directly** – which is what a legal advocate does when she argues a client's case. An advocate cannot be impartial. She must take the part of the person for whom she is advocating.

## FRAMEWORK FOR PRACTICE

A nurse should advocate for her patients:

1. **IF** she is committed to this understanding of nursing.
2. **IF** she is convinced that to do so is a health priority.
3. **IF** she is prepared to carry through her advocacy in order to ensure a significant strengthening of her patient's health (foundations for achievement).
4. **IF** she has undertaken a thorough ethical analysis in order to ensure that her advocacy for this patient will not unreasonably compromise the health of others.

(These **IFS** reflect advocacy's secondary place in the nursing's moral hierarchy.)

The nurse will be helped in her deliberation about whether to advocate if she uses the **Caring Grid** below:

*continues*

*continued*

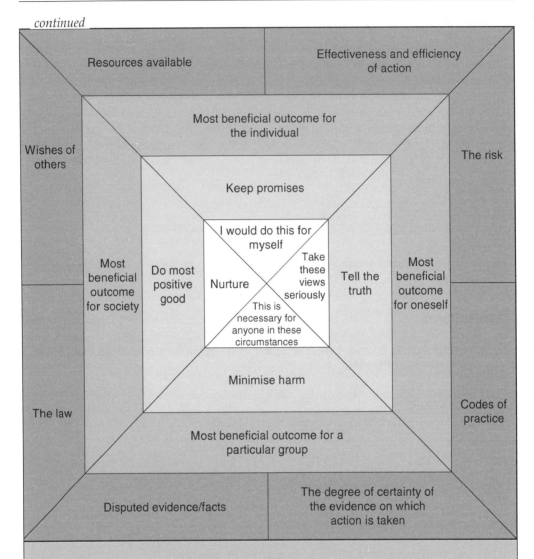

Resources available

Effectiveness and efficiency
of action

Most beneficial outcome for
the individual

Wishes of
others

The risk

Keep promises

I would do this for
myself

Most
beneficial
outcome
for society

Do most
positive
good

Nurture

Take
these
views
seriously

Tell the
truth

Most
beneficial
outcome
for oneself

This is
necessary for
anyone in these
circumstances

Minimise harm

The law

Codes of
practice

Most beneficial outcome for a
particular group

Disputed evidence/facts

The degree of certainty of
the evidence on which
action is taken

The Caring Grid

# PRACTICAL WAYS OF ADVOCATING FOR PATIENTS

It takes experience and practice to use the **Caring Grid** well. Nurses are urged to experiment with it – and any other helpful way to improve their powers of ethical analysis – since the **Universal Code** requires intelligent, practical reflection. **There are neither absolute rules nor binding principles in the ethical realm.**

If a patient has a whim that she ought to have the best bed in the ward – say the one with a pleasant view from the window – a nurse may well decide not to advocate for her on the grounds that her **foundations for achievement** are not unduly damaged by the deprivation, her dignity is intact in her present bed, and

*continues*

_continued_

other patients are equally deserving of the best bed. If, however, a non-dangerous, frail patient is not allowed to push herself around the hospital grounds in a wheelchair – when to do so is the most important expression of autonomy the patient can imagine – then on this understanding of nursing the nurse is likely to want to advocate for her patient.

How she does so will depend on the situation and – perhaps – on her courage. If possible, the nurse who wishes to work for health as a first priority will seek to advocate for a single patient in such as way as to promote the health of many.

## 5. A NURSE SHOULD CARRY OUT RESEARCH IN THE INTERESTS OF THE (ACTUAL OR POTENTIAL) RECIPIENTS OF HER NURSING CARE

A further **secondary purpose of nursing** is to research. The nurse who commits to **foundational nursing** will wish to research honestly, and first and foremost in order to improve the health of actual and potential patients.

### Definition

Research is:

> Any method, applied to any phenomenon, that can produce a greater understanding of that phenomenon.

### FRAMEWORK FOR PRACTICE

The **Honest Researcher Test** should be completed shortly before a nurse prepares a research application, accepts a research grant and begins a research project. The nurse should be open about the results of the **Test** and should be prepared to change her mind as she considers the results. If her proposal is not governed by the **primary set of nursing purposes** she should not proceed with it.

---

## THE HONEST RESEARCHER TEST

### MOTIVATION

A. Why do I want to do this research? 1, 2, 3, 4, 5, 6.
B. What alternative research could I do? a, b, c, etc. i–xiii
C. Will my research find answers that are already well known?
D. I have chosen this research method because: i–vii
E. I will accept and try to publish whatever result I achieve, even if: i–vi
   I am choosing to do this research because ... ...

---

_continues_

*(continued)*

---

**GUIDING PHILOSOPHY**

A. Have I said: 'I am choosing to do this research because I believe its goals are the most important I could possibly aim for?

B. If no, why not?

C. If yes: What are these goals? Are they consistent with nursing values?

D. How likely is it that my research will produce results that will convince others to act in line with nursing values? i–iv

E. Are there better ways open to me to bring about change in line with the goals of nursing I have committed to? . . .

---

## 6. A NURSE SHOULD USE APPROPRIATE METHODS, REASONING AND COMMUNICATION

A further **secondary nursing purpose** is **to use those methods of clinical work, practical and moral reasoning, and communication appropriate to the achievement of the primary nursing tasks**.

It is commonly assumed that this is a **primary nursing purpose**. Yet this is a fundamental mistake[124] – a part of the **Ethics Myth** – and is an assumption that can sometimes cause harm to patients. If **Item 6** is thought to be a primary purpose then – at a stroke – **what happens to be the case** is permitted to set the goals of health care.

For example, if **what is** is allowed to lead the way, then the very presence of therapies or machinery will require their use, whatever the end to which they are used. Only if the notion of **appropriateness** is made subject to **ethically inspired governing tasks** can health care practice be guaranteed to be under humane control. In this case – once it is acknowledged that techniques are useful only in so far as they contribute to the creation of health – **the nurse is liberated**. If she commits to the **Universal Code** she cannot be forced to do something because it is there, rather she can decide to do something if it contributes to the achievement of the other **five items** in this Code. If it does not – or if there are better ways of achieving the **five items** – then she should not do it.

# UNIVERSALITY

Finally, a potentially confusing point must be laid to rest. As explained above, the expression **'Universal Code'** does not mean that the recommendations contained in it are universally right. Nor does it imply that every nurse everywhere **should** obey them. That would be **dictatorial ethics**.

Rather the expression means that **it is possible for any nurse from anywhere living at any time to adopt its values and to apply them constructively in any context in which she finds herself. Any nurse who espouses the values explained in the Code will be able to make good use of it regardless of her (or her patients') culture, historical era or social setting (because she will be promoting health according to the foundations theory)**.

The point can be summarised like this:

1. Any action that might potentially affect another person has **ethical content**.
2. However, how a person chooses to live his life is up to that person – he may or may not choose to make an ethical commitment, and if he does he may commit to an indefinite number of ways of living.
3. **Work for health** is one of these ways of living (at least for part of the ethically committed person's time), and is the basis of the **Universal Code**.
4. Not everyone will want to commit to **work for health** – so the **Code** is not universal in this sense.
5. Not all contexts require **work for health** (a conductor collecting train tickets, a woman washing a car) – so the **Code** is not universal in this sense either.
6. However, since the purpose of nursing is to work humanely for health, it is hard to imagine nurses not wanting to adopt the **Universal Code**.
7. Furthermore, once a nurse has committed to the **Code** she can apply it universally (in the same way to everyone, whatever their culture), as can any other nurse who has adopted it.
8. Note too that the **Code** is not unique to nursing – its universality also lies in the fact that **anyone** who wishes to work kindly for health can use it.

Of course the **Code** will never be universally applied. But it is nevertheless a universal possibility – it **could** be applied universally if every nurse were to accept its values.

Its **additional advantages** are:

1. It is part of a comprehensive understanding of health and ethics, in which work for health and moral analysis are inextricably joined.
2. All its key terms are defined.
3. Different ways of working for health are justified.
4. The nurse is enabled to choose between them according to a clear and logical conceptual hierarchy.
5. The nurse has the choice to commit to this way of thinking or not.
6. It admits that it is not – and cannot possibly be – exclusive to nursing.
7. The **Universal Code** is based on an ethically and practically powerful combination of analytic and nursing philosophy.

## HOW TO USE THE CODE

There are many worked examples in this book. However, there is space for two more to show:

**a. How a nurse might use the Code in her daily work.**
**b. How the Code provides decision-making guidance without dictating answers.**

---

*CASE NINE*

### Domestic Violence

A nurse makes a visit to a house to check on the progress of a three-year-old child. The mother lets the nurse in. The nurse notices that the mother has a black eye, and sees that the child is sitting miserably in a corner, staring at the floor.

---

◆

---

### USING THE CODE IN THIS SITUATION

First, the nurse is not obliged to use the **Universal Code**. She is contracted to a health authority and subject to the law of the land, but whether she chooses to base her practice on the **Code** is up to her. She and only she can decide whether she wishes to make the **ethical commitment** to try to work according to it.

Second, once she has committed to this way of working she can make use of a sturdy, practical framework. Even so, what she does is open to her judgement, within the limits of the theory of health and nursing purpose to which she has committed.

With these points in mind, **the nurse uses the Code as follows**:

1. She asks: **how do I work for health in this situation? How do I apply the foundations understanding of health?**
She has the foundations image in mind. In order to use it properly she has to decide whether the $\hat{\mathbf{I}}$ is an individual or a group – and if so which individual or group. Intuitively, she decides to inspect the foundations first of the mother and then of the child. As she does so she sees that the content of the foundational boxes changes.

She pulls out a blank foundations sheet from a pack she carries with her. The mother knows what to do – she has done this sort of assessment before. Together the nurse and mother describe the current platforms of her and her child (by filling in the empty blocks) – and discuss what to do about those parts that are weakest or missing altogether. **Figures 25** and **26** show how the two pictures look.

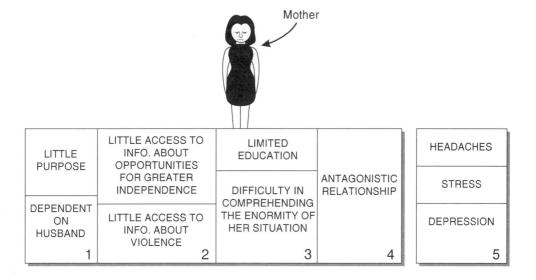

**Figure 25**   The mother's foundations (as they are now)

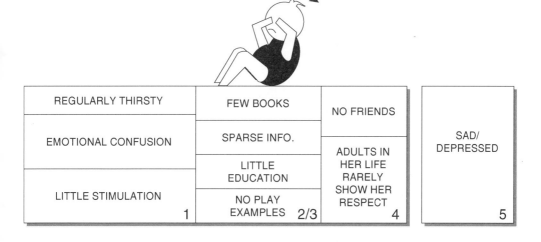

**Figure 26**   The child's foundations (as they are now)

Clearly there are major problems with:

1. The parents' relationship.
2. The mother's life-satisfaction.
3. Lack of information about what the mother might do about a violent husband.
4. The child's emotions (she is confused and sad about her parents' fights).
5. The child's intellectual development (there are no books, computers or explicitly educational toys in the house, and nor does the child play any imaginative games).

**These are the health priorities identified by the nurse.**

2. In order to help her decide which are most fundamental she asks – **do you lack dignity?**
The mother isn't sure what she means so the nurse explains how the Code defines dignity.

'Are you sometimes in circumstances in which you are incapable and in which you feel inadequate?' she asks.

'Yes', the mother replies. 'When he hits me. I don't know what to do. He makes me feel naked.

3. In order to help her decide **in what manner** to offer help to the mother, the nurse reflects: **in what way should I care?**
Of course she is moved by the mother's plight and disturbed by the child's accumulating difficulties – inescapably she is emotionally involved. But should she show it? What form of caring would most promote the health of this woman?

The nurse decides that although she is outraged at the mother's treatment – and feels like screaming and crying with her – she should sympathise and be compassionate but not get any further personally involved. She decides she must keep a professional distance and advise the mother of her options, help her think through the pros and cons of each, and then support her in her decision – whatever it is and whether or not she agrees with it (one consequence of committing to the **foundations theory of health**).

The mother decides she cannot go to the police on her own. She asks the nurse to go with her and – initially at least – help her make her case.

The nurse has to think about this carefully – she has to undertake an **ethical analysis** using the **Caring Grid**. Eventually she decides that three central boxes apply. She

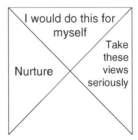

chooses to make the box **maximise benefit for a particular group** her priority, defining the group as the mother and child and defining benefit as 'the chance for them to live a fulfilled life'. She recognises the many **risks** – to the mother, the child, the family and perhaps even to herself, but in this case she opts for the box **do most positive good** rather than **minimise harm**. In this case the latter box seems to advise a cautionary word to the father, whereas the former is more likely to prompt fundamental and – she hopes – positive change.

(Note that the **Caring Grid** analysis can be done at any point – since **ethics is everywhere** and since the Grid asks you to work for health – by using its central boxes.)

She concludes that she ought to advocate – that she should:

> **Speak on behalf of some other person (or persons), as that person perceives her interests**

by going to the police station with the mother.

In this case **Items 5** and **6** of the **Code** are either not relevant or taken as read. Naturally she has tried to make sure her research into this case has been as thorough as possible, but otherwise **Items 1–4** offer her sufficient guidance.

———————— ◆ ————————

This final – very difficult – example is based on a situation in which I was involved. It is included because it highlights how ethically demanding it can be to make nursing decisions in real life – much more is needed than is offered by the usual Codes of Practice. It also reinforces the argument of **Chapter Eight: Mental Health**, that nursing should make its principles theoretically and practically explicit – and stand by them – pressing collectively for change in those areas of mental health care where they do not currently apply. Nursing can do this by courageously adopting the **Universal Code**.

---

## CASE TEN

### Liane

Liane is an obese 34-year-old New Zealander. Her mother is English, her father was French. Liane has her father's olive skin, and despite no Melanesian ancestry is regularly mistaken for a Maori or Pacific Islander.

Liane is intelligent and articulate, yet few can see beyond her volatility. Her fearsome determination to get what she thinks she deserves has never won many friends.

*continues*

— continued —

She has had numerous temporary jobs on the fringe of the music industry, but never a permanent one. She hopes eventually to qualify as a sound engineer and to work in America.

Liane had a music tutor called Jason. According to Jason, Liane had been stalking him for weeks and had written threatening letters. He says she turned up at his college, threw stones at his classroom window, started to undo nuts from his car wheels and yelled abuse at him when he asked her to go.

Liane admits she was attracted to Jason, though she says he deliberately led her on. She did throw stones but took just one nut from one wheel of his car. He stopped her loosening any more by coming at her with a baseball bat. She says she wrestled with him to stop him hitting her.

Indisputably Liane wrote some 40 letters to Jason. They mostly read like love letters from a 14-year-old with a crush, though a handful are angry with him for ignoring her. Jason had previously complained to the police about these letters. Despite the fact Liane had no criminal record or history of mental illness at the time, Jason was believed immediately.

The police arrested Liane and took her to court cells, whereupon she became loudly distressed. As a result she was seen by a psychiatrist who admitted her – against her wishes – to a clinic for assessment and treatment.

In the fortnight between her admission and court appearance things got worse for Liane. She told staff she had psychic powers, could read minds, could affect the future, and needed to find out if Jason was her 'chosen one'. This, she said, is what some witches do.

Liane appeared before a District Court in October 1995, to face 35 charges of 'intent to intimidate', one of 'use of insulting words', one of 'interfering with a motor vehicle', one of 'possessing an offensive weapon' and one of 'threatening to kill'.

She was found guilty of the criminal charges and committed to a mental institution under the **Criminal Justice Act**.

Two years later and Liane was still confined and receiving compulsory medication.

A series of psychiatrists have now declared that Liane is mentally disordered and a danger to herself and others, but they do not agree about what's wrong with her.

Her initial diagnosis was *erotmania*. She has also been said to have:

a bipolar disorder
schizophrenia
a schizo-affective disorder
a mood disorder
antisocial, borderline personality traits
depression

And she has been told by one psychiatrist that he does not consider her mentally ill,

— continues —

*continued*

## DRUG TREATMENTS

During her incarceration Liane has been compelled to take haloperidol, chlorpromazine, benztropine, pimozide, risperidone, fluoxetine (Prozac) and olanzapine. All are anti-psychotics except fluoxetine (an antidepressant) and benztropine, which is given for the treatment of Parkinsonism and drug-induced extra-pyramidal reactions – of which Liane has suffered several, including nausea and vomiting, restlessness, a stiff jaw, tremor, amenorrhoea (from haloperidol), sedation and postural hypotension (from chlorproma-zine), lactation without pregnancy, tardive dyskinesia (from pimozide), ECG changes (from pimozide and haloperidol) and severe chest pain (risperidone).

Not one of these drugs has changed Liane's beliefs in any respect – she maintains today exactly what she said when she first entered the Clinic. She is a witch.

◆

According to the **Ethics Myth**: Liane's psychiatrists and nurses (and the cultural and educational systems that support them) are at **Point X** on the iceberg. They inhabit a mundane world and cannot see that there are any ethical issues in their everyday work. They merely have conventional jobs to do and normal lives to lead when it is time to go home.

But according to the view that the social world **IS** the ethical realm (see **Figure 24**) things are quite different. **Nothing** that is done to Liane or any other patient is ethically neutral.

In every patient's case, beneath the tip of the iceberg there are endless ethical issues for everyone involved – and not least for Liane's nurses. Among other things they should ask: Is there such a thing as mental illness? Is witchcraft a genuine religion? What is a genuine religion? Does one person have a moral right to medicate another against her wishes? To what extent do pharmaceutical companies' business interests impact on the treatment of psychiatric patients?

Such questions are constantly there – whether or not they are visible.

More fundamentally still, for every nurse involved in Liane's case there are never-ending personal ethical questions: What should I say to her? Should I ever restrain her physically? Should I befriend her? Should I keep a professional distance? Should I advocate for Liane against the system? How should I act at work? How should I live?

◆

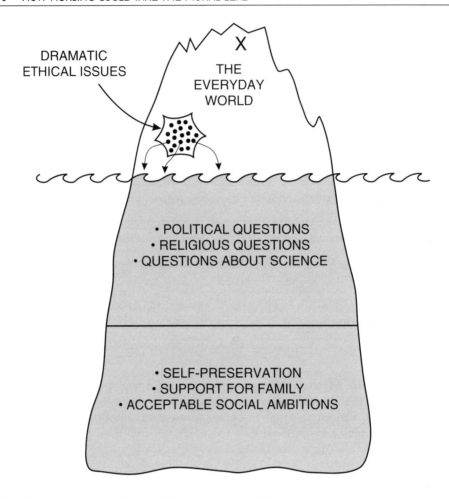

**Figure 22** The moral world according to the Ethics Myth

Now let's consider how a nurse might use the **Universal Code** to work out how to practise.

It is now the present day – two and half years since Liane's arrest for allegedly intimidating Jason. She is still on anti-psychotic medication (olanzapine) and still adamant she is a witch (and indeed that she has always been a witch, in all her past lives). The psychiatrists have just about exhausted their medication options, but are nevertheless as convinced as ever (possibly even more than ever) that she is insane.

However, with typical resourcefulness, Liane has talked them into a deal – a written contract no less. She has agreed to take the olanzapine if they give her home leave. Her consultant has reluctantly – and ambiguously – agreed to this and Liane has been let out for the occasional night, but only on condition she stays with her mother and does not drive. The psychiatrist has also made it very clear that he can lock her up whenever he decides.

It is 9.30 Thursday morning, and time for the 'community meeting' in the Unit. Liane is standing up, straight and assertive, despite her physical bulk. She is asking for weekend leave, explaining why she wants it and what she intends to do.

She is told there will be a decision by Friday lunchtime. She sits down. Then she gets up again and says – can I go swimming next week? She is informed that she must make a written request.

It's 10.30 now and Liane is speaking to Lorraine – one of the nurses.

'When am I going to be discharged?' she asks.

Lorraine says, 'That depends how you behave and what you say about being a witch, doesn't it? When we think it's time for a discharge we will let you know.'

Lorraine carries on, 'We weren't very impressed with you this week so I doubt you'll get leave this weekend, by the way. Get any worse and we might be looking at seclusion again, Dr Simpson might put you on section 57 . . .'

'What's that?' Liane asks.

'It's in the Mental Health Act.'

'Can I see it?'

'We don't hold any copies here, Liane, the Act is for us not you,' Lorraine tells her.

———————— ◆ ————————

An hour later Liane is sitting with a new patient on the Unit, Hinemoa Peters.

'You'll get used to the bastards,' Liane tells her, characteristically. 'Do what you're told and they might let you go in a few weeks – make a fuss like me and they'll fight you all the way to hell.'

'Why have I got to wear pyjamas?' says Hine. 'I'm not sick.'

'It's to keep you down. It's not *for* you. Nothing here is *for* you.'

———————— ◆ ————————

You are a relatively junior nurse on the Unit. You have overheard both conversations and you know that these are typical events. You have also come to the following opinion, over the 18 months you have known of Liane's situation.

You believe:

1. **That Liane's reasons for her actions are not only being disregarded, they are taken as evidence of mental disorder when they are cogent, if you accept her premises.**

2. That she has held her beliefs consistently, coherently and adamantly throughout her detention and treatment, and for most of her life beforehand.
3. That her beliefs are part of a family, cultural and religious tradition of witchcraft.
4. That medication will not and cannot shift these beliefs any more than it could change deep-seated beliefs held by people considered to be mentally normal.
5. That medication and detention have damaged her physically, mentally, socially and financially and will continue to do so until it is halted.
6. That she could not reasonably be considered dangerous to anyone.
7. That she is being held in breach of sections of the Mental Health Act that prohibit detention and treatment solely on religious and cultural grounds.

Thus it is no small matter that you are nursing Liane.


## USING THE CODE IN THIS SITUATION – WORKING FOR LIANE'S HEALTH

Again, you (the nurse) are not obliged to use the **Universal Code**. You are contracted to a health authority and subject to the law of the land – but whether you choose to base your practice on the **Code** is up to you.

However, if you do commit to work according to this code then you **might use it as follows**:

You might first ask: how do I work for health in this situation? By so doing you will be trying to apply the holistic understanding of health defined at **Item 1**. You will also have the Foundations image in mind. In order to use it properly you will have to decide whether the **î** is an individual or a group – and if so which individual or group.

In this case you decide that the image is Liane – no one else. So you need to understand how the image looks in Liane's case.

However, there are two contradictory images – that created by the system and your own and Liane's.


## THE SYSTEM'S IMAGE

Because they have fallen for the **Ethics Myth** and because they have no idea what mental health might be – Liane's stage looks something like **Figure 27** to the psychiatrists (though they do not really think of it in a **Foundational** way).

Box One – she needs medication, she needs to be detained in a secure place, she needs to stop thinking that she is a witch, she needs to accept that she is mentally ill.

Box Two – she doesn't need information, and she certainly does not need books on witchcraft (these are banned). She does not need to see the Mental Health Act.

Box Three – she needs to understand that she is mentally ill. She does not need support in interpreting the Mental Health Act.

Box Four – she does not fit in with the other patients. She needs to learn how to, but there is not much we can do to help her do this.

Box Five – she needs psychiatric therapy until her psychosis goes or is manageable.

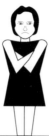

| DRUGS | NO MENTAL HEALTH ACT | COOKING | SHOULD CONFORM TO GROUP NORMS | PSYCHIATRY |
|---|---|---|---|---|
| ACCEPT ILLNESS | NO BOOKS ON WITCHCRAFT | ACCEPT ILLNESS | NEEDS TO FIT IN | PSYCHIATRY |
| DETENTION 1 | OBEY 2 | CRAFTS 3 | SHOULD ACCEPT THE RULES 4 | PSYCHIATRY 5 |

**Figure 27**  Liane's foundations (as they are now) according to the psychiatrists

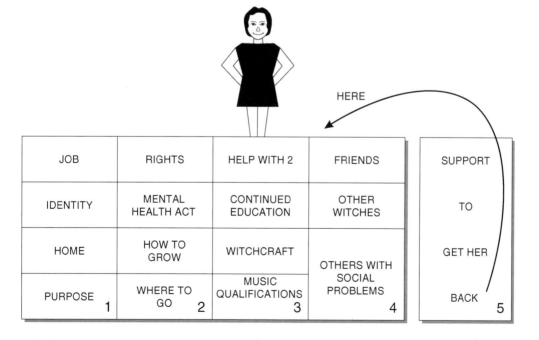

| JOB | RIGHTS | HELP WITH 2 | FRIENDS | SUPPORT |
|---|---|---|---|---|
| IDENTITY | MENTAL HEALTH ACT | CONTINUED EDUCATION | OTHER WITCHES | TO |
| HOME | HOW TO GROW | WITCHCRAFT | OTHERS WITH SOCIAL PROBLEMS | GET HER |
| PURPOSE 1 | WHERE TO GO 2 | MUSIC QUALIFICATIONS 3 | 4 | BACK 5 |

**Figure 28**  A simple view of Liane's foundational/health needs (what she needs to escape her present predicament)

How does Liane's health look like according to the foundations theory humanely understood? How do you – a nurse who wishes to work according to the **Universal Code** – see it?

**Figure 28** offers a graphic view of Liane's health needs. More explicitly:

---

### BOX ONE

She needs a sense of purpose and to have it acknowledged

She needs a job

She needs to be awake and not sedated

She needs to avoid tardive dyskinesia

She needs to be a witch

She needs to get out of the Unit

---

### BOX TWO

She needs to know how to move on

She needs to know her rights

She needs to know how to get help from the outside

---

### BOX THREE

She needs help in interpreting her rights

She needs education programmes in subjects that she will be able to build on

She needs to know more about witchcraft

---

### BOX FOUR

She needs to meet other witches

She needs genuine friends

She needs to know that to be liked one does not have to boast and strut all the time

She needs to see other people with other problems and perhaps to be encouraged to help them

---

### BOX FIVE

She does not need any crisis support – and certainly not any medication – because that crisis is over.

---

You can see that there is a glaring mismatch between these two images. They are so different that at first sight it seems hard to see how you can continue to practise at the Clinic.

However, since you have **committed to work for health** you have a duty to do what you can. In the first place this means working on those foundations it is immediately possible to change, and which you have some power to change.

You are working in a system which is doing things to Liane that you do not believe are work for health. You are a part of it. You even have to make sure that she takes her medication some days.

But you can, at the same time:

1. **Acknowledge that she is a witch.**
2. **Explain her legal rights.**
3. **Provide her with a copy of the Mental Health Act.**
4. **Provide her with 'phone numbers of organisations – including witchcraft associations – that may be able to help her.**
5. **Encourage her to take as many general educational programmes as she can.**

## LIANE'S DIGNITY

In order to help you and her decide which of these are the most fundamental priorities – and to check out exactly where the Code tells you to draw the line between acceptable and unacceptable treatment – you ask – does Liane lack dignity?

In other words you are asking:

**Is Liane in a situation where her capabilities can be effectively applied?**

You can do no other than conclude that she is not. And the reason she is not is to do with the daily practice of the system of which you are a part.

She has to ask for weekend leave in public. She needs an appointment to go swimming. She is patronised by some of the other staff. If she misbehaves she is placed in seclusion and she has to wear pyjamas again. None of these practices are remotely therapeutic yet they go unquestioned by most of the staff. Worse, they seem to be designed to undermine patient dignity.

Rather than act to bring Liane (and other inmates) to above **Line B** on **Figure 6**, part of what the Unit routinely does is to pull Liane down – below the line, to a place where she does not have full dignity.

Given this – and given your commitment to the **Universal Code** – you have to do something to improve this state of affairs. Now you see the situation for what it is, it is not something you can let pass by any longer.

## CARING FOR LIANE

As you decide what to do you must continue to care for Liane. Recalling the diagram of the different ways of caring (**Figure 3** in this book), you recognise that you cannot continue to pursue those 'traditional health service activities' that are undermining Liane's dignity, and nor do you wish to be a part of treatment that is not enhancing – and may be damaging – her foundational health. So, you **cannot** care in this way (**Type B**).

There are further questions: should you care by having a direct personal involvement with Liane (**Type A**) (you do feel strongly that she is being wronged), and should you be prudent and efficient (**Type C**) (taking care in another way)?

You recognise that the answer to both these questions depends on your purpose. You have committed to working for Liane's health first. You consider that though it might be good to befriend her, that this could get in the way of your health work. So you decide to keep an emotional distance.

The question then is – **to what ends should you be prudent and efficient?** You have already rejected some of the Unit's ends. You decide that your ends are:

**a. To bolster Liane's health.**
**b. To ensure that she at least has full dignity.**
**c. To create a more therapeutic environment in the Unit.**

## ADVOCATING FOR LIANE

Should you advocate for Liane? It is an option, but it is a risky one, for both Liane and yourself. There are alternatives – internal protest, external protest, recourse to law, enlisting help from your colleagues, enlisting help from your Union. But each of these is likely to fail against such a well-established system, and may cause more harm than good.

## SO WHAT SHOULD YOU DO?

It is a complicated situation, so you decide to analyse it explicitly – using the **Caring Grid**.

You decide to test out a specific hypothesis: **I should advocate for Liane.** You use the Grid carefully. You itemise the many risks, some of which conflict. There are risks to you, to other patients, to Liane and to the Unit (either way – Liane is in danger if she continues to be treated like this and may also be in danger – of being a scapegoat, of receiving yet more aggressive treatment as a response – if you openly side with her). **Which risks are justified?** you want to know.

You check out the green level of the Grid – **who is your priority?** The safest option is to decide that you should first seek to maximise benefit for yourself, but this would mean going along with not working for Liane's health and dignity (as you interpret it) and you have already decided not to accept this any more.

The most direct option – and the one you have committed to by placing Liane (rather than anyone else) on your Foundations image – is **to try to maximise benefit first for Liane**.

The question then is: **what benefit are you trying to maximise?**

You answer this by asking Liane to define benefit. What does she want most? She says she is dying in this place and must get out – so that is what you decide. To work to have Liane discharged – in the knowledge that your efforts may backfire on you.

You justify your decision on the ground that you have a duty to work for health. Your role as a nurse – you say – is:

---

**To nurture**
**To take Liane's views seriously**
**To help Liane because this is what you would do for yourself**

---

And you believe that escaping a negative regime would be:

---

**Necessary for anyone in these circumstances.**

---

But you have noted some considerable risks so you decide also to abide by the **Universal Code's** fifth point.

> **A nurse should carry out research in the interests of the actual or potential recipients of her nursing care.**

You decide you must get help. You need to take advice about the best way to proceed, in order to minimise harm. You decide that you cannot advocate personally for Liane, because of the many dangerous implications to which this would give rise. However, you can brief other people – patients' associations, medical ethics institutes, human rights organisations, lawyers and so on – who are less vulnerable than you.

You also decide there is far too much silence and collusion in the place, so you raise all the issues that give you cause for concern – in writing, in a professional manner, constructively and persistently.

You ask: why must patients wear pyjamas? How does this dignify them? What is the point of having stressed and easily rattled patients publicly explain their motives? How many anti-psychotics does it take to establish whether a person is truly deluded? What will Liane have to do for the psychiatric system to acknowledge she is cured?

You act – in a small way – to try to change the culture of the institution by asking calm questions about the purpose of the Unit.

You also use your Code in an explicitly positive way – as an educational device. You circulate copies of it to all staff and patients. You ask for time to be set aside regularly to discuss its meaning, and to explore how nurses, care assistants and doctors might apply it in their work.

--------------- ◆ ---------------

The **Universal Code** – like any other set of ideas about how human beings should behave – does not produce perfect answers and may even be used by different nurses to justify dissimilar courses of action. For example, a different nurse might decide she must advocate for Liane, despite the risk. Another nurse might have judged that it would be safer to work gently with Liane and the psychiatrists to get her released into the community, and take it slowly from there.

However, to use the **Code** is to make a solid – and often very specific – commitment to working for a holistic understanding of health, promoting dignity, caring intelligently, advocating for those who cannot speak for themselves, and doing so in a manner that makes good and proper use of the countless techniques and therapies that can be helpful – in the right hands, used for the right reasons.

To use the **Code** like this is to be aware of limits to nursing (and health work) – it is to know specifically where to draw the line. If health is not being created, if a person is being made undignified, if people are not being thoughtfully cared for, and if nurses are staying silent when they see these things – then that is against the **Universal Code**. And it is possible for any nurse – anywhere – to be against these things and for the **Code** – which she will interpret in the cultural and practical context in which she must nurse.

It might be objected that the **Universal Code** is impractical. It might be said that the **Code** spelled out is too complicated, that nurses don't have the time to think like this, that most nurses are not interested in thinking like this, that nurses are not encouraged to think like this, that they are not capable of thinking like this: that nurses neither want nor need the **Universal Code**.

This is undoubtedly partly true – this is what some nursing is like at the moment. But it does not have to be like this – it is possible to change the culture of nursing (after all, nursing is not the same as it was 50 years ago) and equally possible for nursing to change other health care cultures – given the effort and the will.

Furthermore, if these are objections to the **Universal Code** then they are objections to any other ethical strategies meant to be applied meaningfully. Indeed they are objections to the ethically committed, intelligent analysis of health care *per se*.

Nursing simply cannot accept these objections. It is nursing's task to show less tender health workers how to combine kindness and clarity. Ethically sound, practically effective health care must become the norm. The **Universal Ethical Code** is one means of making this happen.

# References

1. Draper, P. (1990). The development of theory in British nursing: current position and future prospects. *J. Advanced Nursing*, **15**, 12–15.
2. International Code of Medical Ethics of the World Medical Association (1949). World Medical Association Bulletin, **1**(3) (October), 109–111.
3. Australian Nursing Council Code of Ethics for Nurses in Australia (May 1993). Value Statement 6.
4. Canadian Nurses Association Code of Ethics for Nursing (adopted in 1985). Canadian Nursing Association, Ottawa.
5. Seedhouse, D.F. (1994). Health care values or business values? *Health Care Analysis*, **2**, 181–186.
6. Seedhouse, D.F. (1994). *Fortress NHS: A Philosophical Review of the National Health Service*, John Wiley, Chichester.
7. Seedhouse, D.F. (1997). *Health Promotion: Philosophy, Prejudice and Practice*, John Wiley, Chichester.
8. British Medical Association. Professional and Scientific Division (1988). *Rights and Responsibilities of Doctors*, London.
9. Smith, R. (1988). All changed, changed utterly. *British Medical Journal*, **316**, 1917–1918.
10. UNESCO, World Health Organisation (1996). *Culture and Health, Orientation Texts on the 1996 Theme*, UNESCO, Paris.
11. Brown J., Kitson, A. and McKnight, T. (1992). *Challenges in Caring: Explorations in Nursing and Ethics*, London, Chapman and Hall.
12. Hover-Kramer, D. (1990). Energy fields: Implications for the science of human caring. NSNA/IMPRINT (Sept./Oct.), pp. 81–82.
13. Holt, J. (1998). The unexamined life is not worth living. In S.D. Edwards (ed.), *Philosophical Issues in Nursing*, London, Macmillan Press, p. 149.
14. Russell, B. (1912). *The Problems of Philosophy*, Oxford University Press, Oxford, London.
15. Seedhouse, D.F. (1998). The paradigm shift X–Y. In *Ethics: The Heart of Health Care*, John Wiley, Chichester, pp. 26ff.
16. UKCC (1996). *Guidelines for Professional Practice*, UKCC.
17. From Lewis Carroll (1871). *Through the Looking Glass and What Alice Found There*, quoted in Gardener, M. (ed.), *The Annotated Alice*, 1970 edn, Penguin Books, Harmondsworth, pp. 268–269.
18. Carroll, L. *Symbolic Logic and the Game of Logic*, Dover, 1958 edn, p. 165.
19. See the *Shorter Oxford English Dictionary*.
20. Curtin, L. (1986). The nurse as advocate: A philosophical foundation for nursing. In Peggy L. Chinn (ed.), *Ethical Issues in Nursing*, Aspen Systems Corporation, Maryland.
21. Heubel, F. (1996). Moral strangers and the health care market. *Health Care Analysis*, **4**, 197–205.
22. Gadow, S. (1983). Existential advocacy: philosophical foundation of nursing. In C.P. Murphy and H. Hunter (eds), *Ethical Problems in the Nurse–Patient Relationship*, Allyn & Bacon, Boston, pp. 40–58.
23. Arnold, E. (1997). Caring from the graduate student perspective. *International Journal for Human Caring*, **1**(3), 32–42.

24. Crowden, A. (1995). Beyond advocacy: further reflections on the moral nature of nursing practice, The Proceedings of the Conference *Impossible Demands: Ethical and Legal Quandaries for Nurses*, Friday 13th October 1995, Monash University Centre for Human Bioethics, ed. John McKie, pp. 97–109.

25. Kerridge, J., Lowe, M. and McPhee, J. (1998). *Ethics and Law for the Health Professions*, Social Science Press, Wentworth Falls, USA. (Here quoting: Sellin, S.C. (1995). Out on a limb: a qualitative study of patient advocacy in institutional nursing. *Nurs. Ethics*, **2**(1), 19–29.)

26. Ingelfinger, F.J. (1980). Arrogance. *New England Journal of Medicine*, **303**, 1507–1511.

27. Copi, Irving M. (1953). *Introduction to Logic*, Macmillan, New York.

28. Barnum, B.S. (1998). *Nursing Theory: Analysis, Application, Evaluation*, 5th edn, Lippincott, Philadelphia.

29. Johnstone, M.-J. (1994). *Bioethics*, 2nd edn, Sydney, W.B. Saunders/Baillière Tindall.

30. Leininger, Madeleine M. (ed.) (1990). *Ethical and Moral Dimensions of Care*, Wayne State University Press, Detroit.

31. Knowlden, V. (1990). The virtue of caring in nursing. In Madeleine M. Leininger (ed.), *Ethical and Moral Dimensions of Care*, Wayne State University Press, Detroit.

32. Mayeroff, M. (1971). *On Caring*, Harper and Row, London.

33. Watson, J. (1985). *Nursing: Human Science and Human Care. A Theory of Nursing*, Appleton–Century–Crofts, Norwalk, CT. Cited in Fry, S.T. (1990). The philosophical foundations of caring, in Leininger, *Ethical and Moral Dimensions of Care*.

34. Watson, J. (1990). The moral failure of the patriarchy. *Nursing Outlook*, **38**(2), 62–66.

35. Watson, J. (1989). Human caring and suffering: a subjective model for health sciences. In *They Shall Not Hurt: Human Suffering and Human Caring*, ed. R. Taylor and J. Watson, Colorado Associated University Press.

36. Taylor, R. and Watson, J. (1989). *They Shall Not Hurt: Human Suffering and Human Caring*, Colorado Associated University Press.

37. Reed, J. (1994). Two paradoxes of caring: a response to Gorovitz. *Health Care Analysis*, **2**(3), 217–220.

38. Noddings, N. (1984). *Caring: A Feminine Approach To Ethics and Moral Education*, University of California Press, Berkeley, CA.

39. Ray, M. (1980). A philosophical analysis of caring within nursing. *First National Conference: The Phenomena and Nature of Caring*, Salt Lake City, Utah.

40. Pellegrino, E. (1985). The caring ethic: the relation of physician to patient. In *Caring, Curing, Coping: Nurses, Physician, Patient Relationships*, ed. A.H. Bishop & J.R. Scudder, University of Alabama Press, pp. 8–30.

41. Health Advisory Service (1999). *'Not because they are old' An independent inquiry into the care of older people on acute wards in general hospitals*, Health Advisory Service 2000.

42. Help the Aged (1999). *The Dignity on the Ward Manual – How to improve hospital care for older people*, Help the Aged, London.

43. Baker, Dorothy E. (1983). 'Care' in the geriatric ward: An account of two styles of nursing. In J. Wilson-Barnett (ed.), *Nursing Research: Ten Studies in Patient Care*, Wiley, Chichester, pp. 108–109.

44. Australian Nursing Council (1993). *Code of Ethics for Nurses in Australia*. Australian Nursing Council July 1993, Canberra. See: (Shotton, L.) and Seedhouse, D. (1998). Practical dignity in caring. *Nursing Ethics*, **5**(3), 246–255.

45. Australian Nursing Council (July 1995). *Code of Professional Conduct for Nurses in Australia*, Australian Nursing Council, Canberra. See: (Shotton, L.) and Seedhouse, D. (1998). Practical dignity in caring. *Nursing Ethics*, **5**(3), 246–255.

46. Commonwealth Standards for Nursing Homes (1987). *Objective 4.1*, Australian Government Publishing Service, Canberra. See: (Shotton, L.) and Seedhouse, D. (1998). Practical dignity in caring. *Nursing Ethics*, **5**(3), 246–255.

47. H.M. Government, UK (1995). *Patient's Charter*, Department of Health, London, p. 6.

48. United Kingdom Central Council for Nurses, Midwives and Health Visitors (1992). *Code of Professional Conduct*, UKCC.

49. Seedhouse, D.F. (September 1991). 'A Right to be Heard', an interview with Graham Pink. *Health Matters*, **8**, 8–9.

50. Mairis, Elaine D. (1994). Concept clarification in professional practice – dignity. *J. Advanced Nursing*, **19**, 947–953, 952.

51. Haddock, Jane (1996). Towards further clarification of the concept 'dignity'. *J. Advanced Nursing*, **24**, 924–931, 930.

52. Department of Health and Family Services, Commonwealth of Australia (1997). *Issues Relating to the Resident Classification Scale*, Canberra, Australian Government Publishing Services, 8–31.

53. Parker, S. (1996). *The Human Body*, Harry N. Abrams, New York.

54. Woods, S. (1998). A theory of holism for nursing. *Medicine, Health Care and Philosophy*, **1**(3), 255–261.

55. Koestler, A. (1979). *Janus: A Summing Up*, Pan Books, London.

56. Hawley, G. (ed.) (1997). *Ethics Workbook for Nurses: Issues, Problems and Resolutions*, Social Science Press, Wentworth Falls, USA, p. 6.

57. Kerridge, J., Lowe, M. and McPhee, J. (1998). *Ethics and Law for the Health Professions*, Social Science Press, Wentworth Falls, USA.

58. Gillon, R. (1992). Caring, men and women, nurses and doctors, and health care ethics. *J. Med. Ethics*, **18**, 171–172.

59. Gallagher, A. (1995). Medical and nursing ethics: never the twain? *Nursing Ethics*, **2**(2), 95–101.

60. Nieswiadomy, R.M. (1998). *Foundations of Nursing Research*, 3rd edn, Appleton and Lange, Stamford, Connecticut.

61. Polit, D.F. and Hungler, B.P. (1995). *Nursing Research: Principles and Methods*, 5th edn, J.B. Lippincott, Philadelphia.

62. Wilson, H.S. (1985). *Research in Nursing*, Addison-Wesley, Reading, MA.

63. Seaman, C.C.H. and Verhonick, P.J. (1982). *Research Methods for Undergraduate Students in Nursing*, Appleton–Century–Crofts, New York.

64. Fox, D.J. (1982). *Fundamentals of Research in Nursing*, 4th edn, Appleton–Century–Crofts, New York.

65. Krampitz, S.D. and Pavlovich, N. (1981). *Readings for Nursing Research*, C.V. Mosby Co., St Louis, MO.

66. Seedhouse, D.F. (1995). *Reforming Health Care: The Philosophy and Practice of International Health Reform*, John Wiley, Chichester.

67. Rose, S.M. and Black, B.L. (1985). *Advocacy and Empowerment: Mental Health Care in the Community*, Routledge & Kegan Paul, Boston.

68. Teasdale, K. (1999). *Advocacy in Health Care*, Blackwell Science, Malden, Massachusetts.

69. Wolf, Z.R. (1986). Foreword. *Topics in Clinical Nursing*, **8**(2), viii.

70. Sarason, S.B. (1985). *Caring and Compassion in Clinical Practice*, Jossey-Bass, San Francisco, California.

71. Galanti, G.-A. (1991). *Caring for Patients from Different Cultures: Case Studies from American Hospitals*, University of Pennsylvania Press, Philadelphia.

72. Routasalo, P. and Isola, A. (1996). The right to touch and be touched. *Nursing Ethics*, **3**(2), 165–176.

73. Coney, S. (1997). To the uninformed: managed care means damaged ethics. *Health Care Analysis*, **5**(3), 252–258.

74. Seedhouse, D.F. (1997). Tautology and value: the flawed foundations of health economics. *Health Care Analysis*, **5**(1), 1–5.

75. Jadad, A.R. (ed.) (1998). *Randomised Controlled Trials: A User's Guide*, BMJ Books, London.

76. Lutzen, K. (1997). Nursing ethics into the next millennium: a context-sensitive approach for nursing ethics. *Nursing Ethics*, **4**(3), 219.

77. Gilligan, C. (1982). *In a Different Voice: Psychological Theory and Women's Development*, Harvard University Press, Cambridge, MA.

78. Davis, D.S. (1985). Nursing: an ethic of caring. *Hum. Med.*, **2**, 19–25.

79. Nortvedt, P. (1998). Sensitive judgement: an inquiry into the foundations of nursing ethics. *Nursing Ethics*, **5**(5), 385–392.

80. McCance, T.V., McKenna, H.P. and Boore, J.R.P. (1997). Caring: dealing with a difficult concept. *Int. J. Nurs. Stud.*, **34**(4), 241–248.

81. Jameton, A. (1984). *Nursing Practice: The Ethical Issues*, Prentice-Hall, Englewood Cliffs, NJ.

82. Allmark, P. (1995). Can there be an ethics of care? *Journal of Medical Ethics*, **21**, 19–24.
83. Kuhse, H. (1997). *Caring: Nurses, Women and Ethics*, Blackwell, Oxford.
84. Kottow, M.H. (1999). In defence of medical ethics. *Journal of Medical Ethics*, **25**, 340–343.
85. Tooley, M. (1983). *Abortion and Infanticide*, Clarendon Press, Oxford.
86. Scarre, G. (1996). *Utilitarianism*, Routledge, London.
87. Money, G., Jan, S. and Wiseman, V. (1995). Examining preferences for allocating health care gains. *Health Care Analysis*, **3**(3), 261–265.
88. Williams, A. (1995). Health economics and health care priorities. *Health Care Analysis*, **3**(3), 221–234.
89. Farrar, S., Donaldson, D., Macphee, S., Walker, A. and Mapp, T. (1997). Riposte. Creativity and sacrifice: two sides of the coin. A reply to David Seedhouse. *Health Care Analysis*, **5**(4), 306–309.
90. Donaldson, C., Farrar, S., Walker, A., Mapp, T. and Macphee, S. (1997). Assessing community values in health care: is the 'willingness to pay' method feasible? *Health Care Analysis*, **5**(1), 7–29.
91. An anonymous reviewer of the proposal for this book – a Professor of Nursing.
92. Thompson, Ian E., Melia, Kath M. and Boyd, Kenneth M. (1994). *Nursing Ethics*, 3rd edn, Churchill Livingstone, Edinburgh, preface, p. ix.
93. Seedhouse, D.F. (1992). The two languages of care. *J. Advances in Health and Nursing Studies*, **1**(4), 23–32.
94. Davis, J.A. (1990). Are there limits to caring? Conflict between autonomy and beneficence. In Madeleine M. Leininger (ed.), *Ethical and Moral Dimensions of Care*, Wayne State University Press, Detroit, p. 25.
95. Fox, R.M. and DeMarco, J.P. (1990). *Moral Reasoning: A Philosophic Approach to Applied Ethics*, Holt, Rinehart and Winston, Fort Worth, Texas.
96. Watts, A.W. (1962). *The Way of Zen*, Pelican Books, London, p. 55.
97. Seedhouse, D.F. (1997). What's the difference between health care ethics, medical ethics and nursing ethics? *Health Care Analysis*, **5**(4), 267–274.
98. Brody, B.A. and Englehardt, H.T., Jr (eds) (1980). *Mental Illness: Law and Public Policy*, Dordrecht, Holland.
99. Campbell, T. and Heginbotham, C. (1991). *Mental Illness: Prejudice, Discrimination and the Law*. Avebury, Aldershot, Hants.
100. Greenland, C. (1970). *Mental Illness and Civil Liberty: A Study of Mental Health Review Tribunals in England and Wales*, Bell, London.
101. Clinton, M. and Nelson, S. (eds) (1996). *Mental Health and Nursing Practice*, Prentice-Hall, Sydney.
102. American Psychiatric Association (1995). *Diagnostic and Statistical Manual of Mental Disorders*, 4th edn, DSM IV, APA, Washington, DC.
103. Marshall, R. (1990). The genetics of schizophrenia: axiom or hypothesis. In R. Bentall (ed.), *Reconstructing Schizophrenia*, Routledge, London.
104. http://www.mentalhealth.com/drugs/f33-h02.html
105. Sallee, F.R., Nesbitt, L., Jackson, C., Sine, L. and Sethuraman, G. (1997). Relative efficacy of haloperidol and pimozide in children and adolescents with Tourette's disorder. *Am. J. Psychiatry*, **154**(8), 1057–1062.
106. Tollefson, G.D. and Sanger, T.M. (1997). Negative symptoms: a path analytic approach to a double-blind, placebo- and haloperidol-controlled clinical trial with olanzapine. *Am. J. Psychiatry*, **154**(4), 466–474.
107. Lindstrom, E. and von Knorring, L. (1994). Changes in single symptoms and separate factors of the schizophrenic syndrome after treatment with risperidone or haloperidol. *Pharmacopsychiatry*, **27**(3), 108–113.
108. Breggin, P.R. (1994). *Toxic Psychiatry*, St. Martin's Press, New York.
109. United Kingdom Central Council for Nursing and Midwifery (1996). *Guidelines for Mental Health and Learning Disabilities Nursing*, UKCC.
110. Burns, P. (1991). Elements of spirituality and Watson's Theory of Transpersonal Caring: expansion of focus. In P.L. Chinn (ed.), *Anthology on Caring*, National League for Nurses, NY, pp. 141–153.

111. Falloon, R.H. and Fadden, G. (1993). *Integrated Mental Health Care*, Cambridge University Press, New York.
112. Breemer ter Stege, C.P.C. et al (1983). *Mental Health Care in the Netherlands*, Nederlands centrum Geestelijke volksgezonheid, Utrecht.
113. Barker, P., Campbell, P. and Davidson, B. (1999). *From the Ashes of Experience: Reflections on Madness, Survival and Growth*, WHURR, London.
114. Breggin, P.R. (1994). *Toxic Psychiatry*, St. Martin's Press (p. 392, 'What do patients want for themselves?').
115. Tingle, J. and Cribb, A. (eds) (1994). *Nursing Ethics and the Law*, Blackwells, Oxford, p. 172.
116. American Psychiatric Association. Task force on Electroconvulsive Therapy (1978). *Electroconvulsive Therapy*, APA, Washington, DC.
117. American Psychiatric Association (1995). *Diagnostic and Statistical Manual of Mental Disorders*, 4th edn, DSM IV, APA, Washington, DC, p. xxi.
118. Morrall, P. (1998). *Mental Health Nursing and Social Control*, WHURR, London.
119. Owens, R.G. (1985). *Violence: A Guide for the Caring Professions*, Croom Helm, London.
120. Clare, A. (1976). *Psychiatry in Dissent*, Tavistock, London.
121. Seedhouse, D.F. (1986). *Health: The Foundations for Achievement*, John Wiley, Chichester.
122. www.mentalhealth.com
123. Downie, R.S., Fyfe, C. and Tannahill, A. (1990). *Health Promotion: Models and Values*, Oxford University Press, Oxford.
124. Seedhouse, D.F. (1991). *Liberating Medicine*, John Wiley, Chichester.
125. Wesley, Ruby L. (1992). *Nursing Theories and Models*, Springhouse, Springhouse PA.
126. Pearson, A., Vaughan, B. and Fitzgerald, M. (1996). *Nursing Models for Practice*, 2nd edn, Butterworth-Heinemann, Oxford.
127. Parse, R.R. (ed.) (1999). *Illuminations: The Human Becoming Theory in Practice and Research*, Jones and Bartlett, Boston.
128. Rogers, M. (1970). *An Introduction to the Theoretical Basis of Nursing*, F.A. Davis, Philadelphia.
129. Hunick, G. (1995). *Study Guide to Nursing Theories*, Campion Press, Edinburgh.
130. Meleis, A.I. (1997). *Theoretical Nursing: Development and Progress*, 3rd edn, Lippincott–Raven, Philadelphia.
131. Allmark, P. (1998). Is caring a virtue? *J. Advanced Nursing*, **28**(3), 466–472.
132. Scanlon, C. and Glover, J. (1995). A professional Code of Ethics: providing a moral compass for turbulent times. *Oncology Nursing Forum*, **22**(10).
133. Scott, P.A. (1998). Professional Ethics: are we on the wrong track? *Nursing Ethics*, **5**(6), 477–485.
134. American Nurses Association (1994). Revised Position Statement, 'The Nonnegotiable Nature of the ANA Code for Nurses with Interpretive Statements', ANA Center for Ethics and Human Rights.
135. New Zealand Medical Association. *Code of Ethics*, 4th Draft (in preparation).
136. Seedhouse, D.F. (1998). *Ethics: The Heart of Health Care*, John Wiley, Chichester, pp. 128–131.

# Index

Note: page numbers in *italics* refer to figures

*Index compiled by Jill Halliday*

# Claude Monet

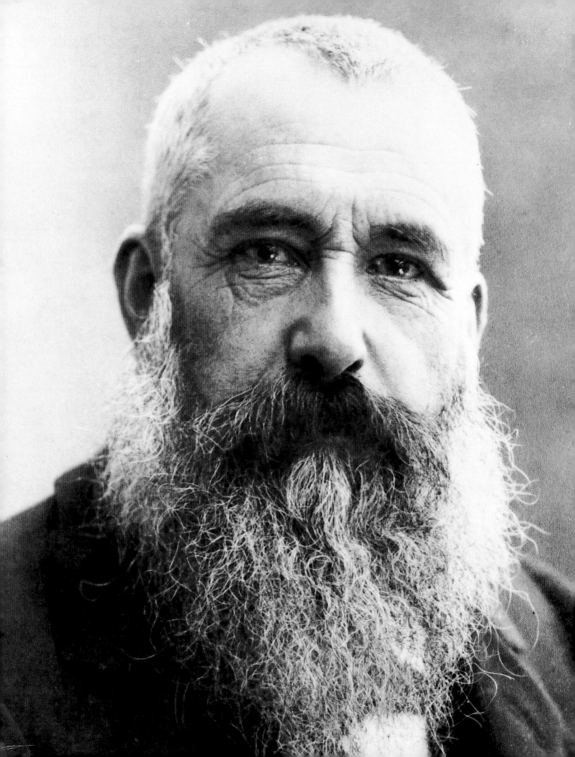